POISONS AND TOXINS

POISONS AND TOXINS

by Joan Arehart-Treichel

HOLIDAY HOUSE · NEW YORK

Printed in the United States of America

Library of Congress Cataloging in Publication Data

Arehart-Treichel, Joan.
Poisons and toxins.

Bibliography: p. 152
Includes index.
SUMMARY: Examines the effects of poisons and toxins from various sources.
1. Poisons—Juvenile literature. 2. Toxins—Juvenile literature. [1. Poisons. 2. Toxins]
I. Title.
RA1213.A73 615.9 76-15034
ISBN 0-8234-0288-6

For Emily and Ben—
who supported my search
for snakes along Elkhorn Creek,
with the exception of water moccasins!

Acknowledgment

I'm grateful to the many toxicologists and other scientists who helped me prepare this book, especially Dr. Phillip Rosenberg of the University of Connecticut School of Pharmacy and editor of *Toxicon*; Dr. Bruce Halstead of Colton, California; Dr. James P. Weston of the University of New Mexico; Dr. Eugene J. Gangarosa of the HEW Center for Disease Control in Atlanta; Dr. Pushkar Kaul of the University of Oklahoma; and Dr. Sherman Minton of Indiana University Medical Center.

Contents

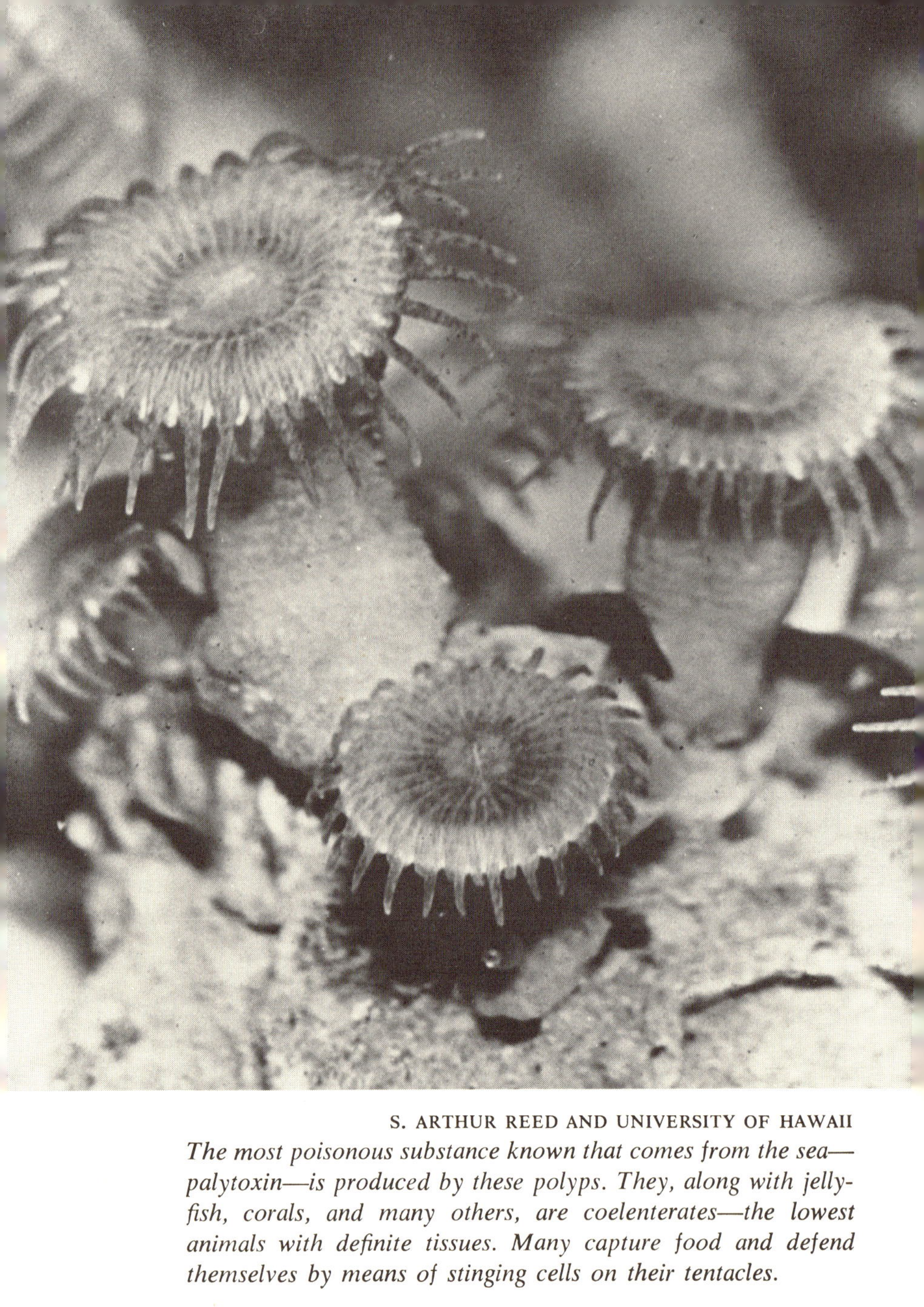

S. ARTHUR REED AND UNIVERSITY OF HAWAII

The most poisonous substance known that comes from the sea—palytoxin—is produced by these polyps. They, along with jellyfish, corals, and many others, are coelenterates—the lowest animals with definite tissues. Many capture food and defend themselves by means of stinging cells on their tentacles.

1 · The Varied World of Poisons

For many years Hawaiians on the island of Maui greatly feared a particular tide pool. They said that it contained a poisonous seaweed and that disaster would strike anyone trying to gather it.

This belief was still very much alive in December 1961. At that time Dr. P. J. Scheuer and his chemistry team at the University of Hawaii set out to discover the mythical tide pool and collect some of its seaweed. Through an elaborate chain of informers, they finally found the right one. But each informer also warned them that misfortune would hit them if they touched the seaweed. In fact, the very afternoon that they took some, a fire destroyed the main building of their laboratory. No ready explanation for the fire could be found. Also, one of the scientists who had scratched his arms and legs while collecting the plant started to feel sick. Apparently a poison from it had entered his body through the scratches.

Nonetheless the scientists carried the seaweed back

to what remained of their lab. They examined it and found that it wasn't seaweed at all. In fact, it wasn't even a plant, but a marine animal that makes a deadly toxin. They and scientists at other universities have since found that it is the most poisonous marine substance known. It is called palytoxin.

This true story about the discovery of palytoxin and the legends and fears that surrounded it underscores the dramatic power that poisons hold over people. Such awe and respect, however, is nothing new. It is as old as the history of humanity.

Back in 4000 B.C., for example, the Mesopotamians had a goddess of potions and poisons. Around 2000 B.C. the Egyptians wrote about puffer fish poison and other toxins, and mentioned the use of charms against snake poison. The Israelis recorded their respect for poisons in the Bible. According to the Book of Exodus 7:19–21: "And the Lord spake unto Moses, Say unto Aaron, Take thy rod, and stretch out thine hand upon the waters of Egypt, upon their streams, upon their rivers, and upon their ponds, and upon all their pools of water, that they become blood; . . . and all the waters that were in the river turned to blood. And the fish that were in the river died; and the river stank, and the Egyptians could not drink of the water of the river; and there was blood throughout all the land of Egypt." This passage is thought to be the earliest record of the toxic effects of the red tide, a condition that comes from billions of protozoa developing at once.

Greeks living from 800 B.C. to 200 B.C. are also known to have had a healthy respect for poisons. In one of his poems, Homer refers to a man bitten by a venomous snake on his journey. By 300 A.D. the people of India were also concerning themselves with treatments for the bites of venomous snakes. And by the year 1000 the Chinese recorded a number of fish with toxic properties—bass, eel, sturgeon, catfish, puffer, stingray. During the Middle Ages in Europe, poisons also probably continued to be feared and respected. But little was written on the subject.

A sharp spine on the tail of this stingray, a curious type of fish, can send poisons into the body of a swimmer who has the misfortune to step on one. The toxins are produced by glands at the base of the spine. The poisonous nature of stingrays was recognized by the Chinese about 1000 years ago.

DR. WALTER A. STARCK II, UNIVERSITY OF MIAMI

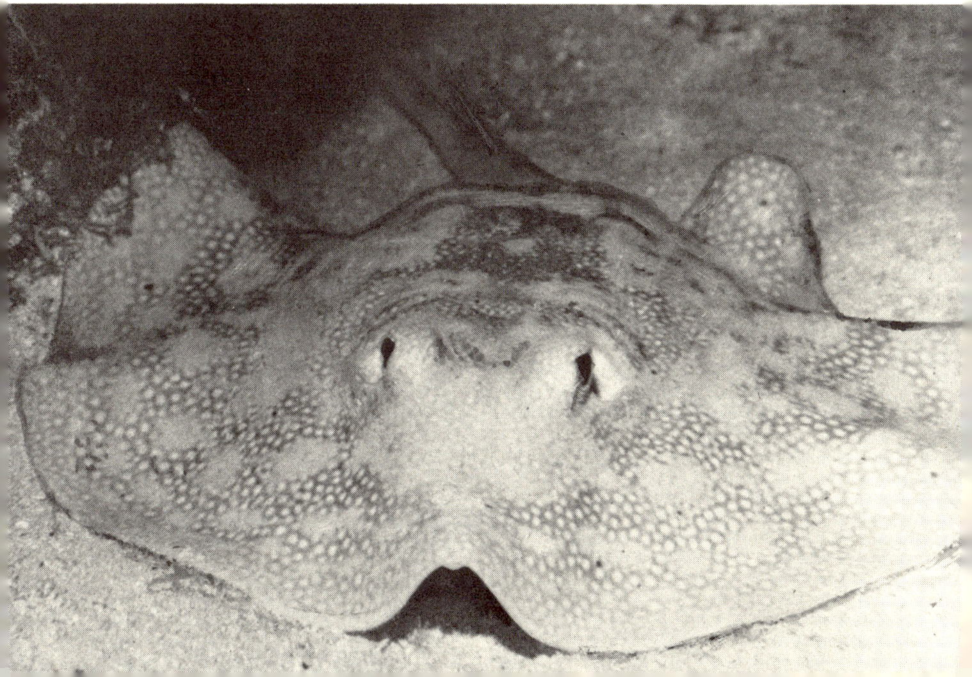

The first reference to a poison in America was made in the fifteenth century in records about Columbus' journeys. It was the poison of the fish in the West Indies causing ciguatera, a toxic illness from eating its flesh. By the sixteenth century educated persons were beginning to take more of a scientific interest in poisons. However, less educated peoples still considered poisonings to be "acts of God."

Throughout history, however, people have not just feared natural poisons. As they have come to learn more and more about them and how they work, they have used them to kill their enemies. In the Greek poem "Cassandra," written in 250 B.C., for example, Cassandra speaks of predicting the death of Ulysses by a spear tipped with the sting of a venomous fish. It was probably a stingray. The early Romans found poisoning such an attractive method for taking life that professional poisoners became the fashion. A famous poisoner at the time was a woman named Locusta. She was a former slave who was pardoned from a death sentence so that she could carry out poisonings thought to be of value to the state. She was even required to train others in her secrets so that they would not be lost upon her death.

A law against criminal poisoning came into effect in Rome in 82 B.C. But it did not deter poisonings. In fact, they flourished in Italy well up into the sixteenth century. The powerful Italian Borgia family was especially adept at poisoning. Cesare Borgia wore a signet ring that contained a secret compartment for arsenic.

Witches and Poisoned Arrows

In other European countries during these centuries, poisoning was also in vogue. Macbeth, an eleventh-century king of Scotland, made a truce with invading Danes and gave them wine spiked with a plant poison. The poison drugged the Danes, then Macbeth had them all slain. Witches used plant poisons to "fly by broomstick" to sabbaths. Actually the poisons made them hallucinate so that they thought they were flying. Some persons put poisons in gloves, letters, books, cutlery, crockery, underclothes, and toothpicks to kill off their enemies. Women even used poisons to rid themselves of no-longer-desirable lovers. They wet their lips with poison, then introduced the poison into the mouths of their victims while kissing them.

When the Europeans discovered America, they found that Americans too could poison. Indians in the Amazon Valley of South America, for instance, were found to kill their enemies with arrows dipped in curare. This is a violent poison that attacks the nerves controlling muscles, paralyzing a victim but leaving his mind clear to recognize his plight. Or as Sir Walter Raleigh described the effect: "Besides the mortality of the wound they make, the party shot endureth the the most insufferable torment in the world, and abideth a most ugly and lamentable death. . . ."

Poisoning as a tool for getting rid of one's enemies continued well into the nineteenth century and beyond. A rascally "holy man" and politician lived in Russia from 1872 to 1916. His name was Rasputin. Once Prince Youssoupoff considered Rasputin to be Russia's most dangerous internal enemy. So he invited him to tea and fed him cakes loaded with the poison potassium cyanide. Rasputin ate lots of the cakes. Usually this poison kills almost instantly, but Rasputin didn't show signs of poisoning until two hours later. Frustrated and alarmed because it was taking so long to kill him, the prince finally shot him.

And indeed, poisoning is no stranger to the twentieth century. Some toxic weapons—tear-gas grenades and chlorine gas—were used during World War I. During the 1975 United States Senate hearings into the activities of the Central Intelligence Agency, it was learned that the CIA had tried, unsuccessfully, to poison Cuba's Premier Castro.

In spite of the negative effects of poisons, some good uses have also been found for them throughout history. Chemicals from plants and animals have been turned into drugs. A number of these chemicals are poisons, such as curare and digitalis, the latter from the foxglove plant. Nonbiological poisons, such as the heavy metals, are also used for positive effects. People living in the Alps in Austria, for example, eat arsenic on a regular basis as a love potion. But the line between how much of a poison is harmful and how much is beneficial is usually small. So an overdose of a poison-based drug can easily kill. In fact, as Dr. Victor diStefano, a pharmacologist at the University of Rochester, warns, "Don't forget that all drugs are poisonous because they are foreign chemicals" in the body.

"Anything Is Poisonous if . . ."

So actually what is a poison? "Anything is poisonous if you give it in large enough amounts," asserts Dr. John Hogg, director of experimental chemistry and biology at the Upjohn Company. Dr. John Adams of the Pharmaceutical Manufacturers Association agrees: "There is such a thing as water intoxication. You can drink too much water and kill yourself; the same with too much sugar, too much salt. It's a question of degree." On the whole, though, scientists tend to agree that the term "poison" is usually reserved for those substances that can kill in very small amounts, whether they are injected by needle, eaten, or absorbed through the skin. In fact, the less of a substance it takes to kill, the more poisonous it is considered to be.

Many natural substances are poisons. There are poisons produced by tiny organisms that cannot be seen except under a microscope. There are those made by plants and animals. Poisons are even made by people. Human saliva contains poisons that closely resemble some toxins in rattlesnake venom, Dr. C. A. Bonilla of Colorado State University has found. He doesn't know of any instance in which a person has killed another person by biting him, but he thinks it is possible. "Most dentists who work with children," he says, "will be the first to tell you that they are afraid of being bitten by children. It has been well known for many years that bites from children are especially toxic." Human menstrual blood also contains some toxic materials. Whether it can do harm remains to be seen.

A number of nonbiological substances in the environment are also poisonous. The heavy metals, as mentioned above, are the major example. According to Dr. J. M. Wood, a biochemist at the University of Illinois, "The natural poisons are undoubtedly the most difficult to study because certain amounts are always present in the environment. Also, a small disturbance in an ecosystem can bring about a natural increase in the rate of synthesis of these compounds. Technically, therefore, it is simpler to monitor the amount of toxic compounds that are synthesized industrially."

Nonetheless there is an incredible number of poisonous synthetic compounds—many more than of the natural ones. Whereas there are thousands of natural poisons, there are hundreds of thousands of synthetic ones, Dr. Phillip Rosenberg of the University of Connecticut School of Pharmacy, and the editor of *Toxicon*, estimates. (*Toxicon* is the major international journal for scientists who study poisons.) Some of these synthetic compounds, such as drugs and household products, were created to help people. Their ability to poison is incidental and undesirable. Other compounds, however, were devised solely to kill. Chemical-warfare poisons and pesticides are two examples.

More and more toxic synthetic materials are being introduced into the environment. Even so, natural poisons still continue to be more harmful. Here is a quick overview of both kinds, proving this point.

POISON	MINIMUM LETHAL DOSE*
botulinus toxin (from a microorganism)	0.00003
tetanus toxin (from a microorganism)	.0001
palytoxin (from a marine animal)	.15
diphtheria toxin (from a microorganism)	.3
cobra toxin (from a snake)	.3
saxitoxin (from a microorganism)	9.0
curare (from a plant)	500.0
strychnine (from a plant)	500.0
dilsopropyl-fluorophosphate (synthetic war gas)	3000.0
sodium cyanide (synthetic poison)	10000.0

* Expressed in $\mu g/kg$, or micrograms per kilogram of body weight. This means that if we are considering saxitoxin, for instance (which has a value of 9.0 micrograms), and the person in question weighs 50 kilograms, it would take at least 50 x 9, or 450 micrograms, of saxitoxin to kill him.

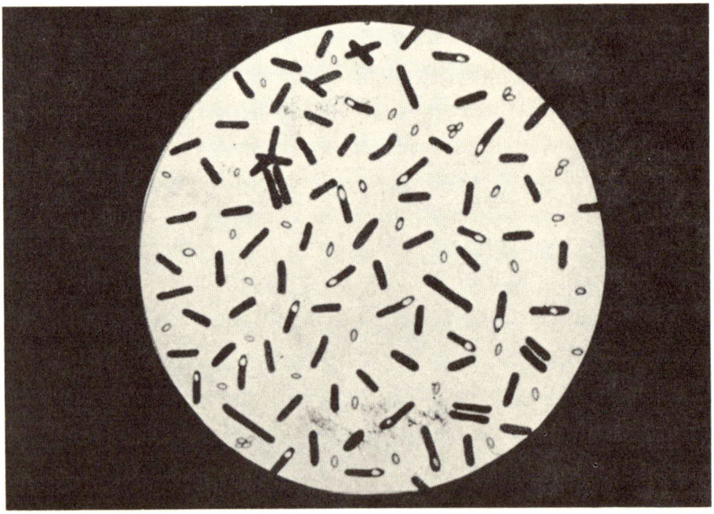

CENTER FOR DISEASE CONTROL, ATLANTA
These are Clostridium botulinum, *the bacteria that produce the food poisoning called botulism. Their toxin is so strong that one researcher calls it "the most fantastic poison that is known."*

It seems ironical that the most poisonous substance in the world—the botulinus toxin, which causes botulism, the most severe food-poisoning killer—is made by a minute organism. (Some scientists have estimated that one ounce of the toxin would be enough to kill 60 million people.) Why is this organism so honored with this world-shaking power? Scientists don't know. But this they're sure of: the key to its toxicity lies in its chemical makeup. As Dr. E. J. Schantz of the University of Wisconsin says, "The toxicity seems to be due to the conformational structure of the protein, because when we distort the conformation of the molecule, it loses its toxicity." In other words, it's the chemical structure of the poison that allows it to attack its victim in a particularly deadly way.

Its deadliness has been expressed very picturesquely by one authority, Dr. Bruce W. Halstead. Referring to its minimum lethal dose, listed first in the table above, he says: "That is almost equivalent to having a flea on a freight car which is 100 miles long, and when the flea gets on, it derails the entire train. This is the most fantastic poison that is known. It is so toxic that it is almost incomprehensible to anyone."

Nerves and Muscles

"It prevents the release of a chemical called acetylcholine at the end of nerves," explains Dr. Eugene J. Gangarosa of the U. S. Department of Health, Education and Welfare's Center for Disease Control in Atlanta. "Without this chemical, nerve conduction doesn't occur. This leads to paralysis of muscles of the diaphragm, and breathing stops. The victim dies by suffocation."

The chemical makeups of all poisons, in fact, are what make them poisons. And their particular makeups are what allow them to damage their victims in highly specific ways. For instance, another potent toxin made by a small organism—the tetanus bacillus—has a different chemical makeup from the botulinus toxin and does just the opposite. It overstimulates nerves in the body, and this leads to muscle spasms, particularly in the jaws. For that reason tetanus is also known as "lockjaw." Because of its particular kind of molecule, arsenic goes for the heart, kidneys, and other organs and irritates the stomach and intestines. Hydrocyanic acid (perhaps better known as prussic acid) keeps oxygen from reaching tissues in the body and also acts on the central nervous system.

Still, certain poisons resemble each other chemically, at least to some degree. Toxins produced by microorganisms tend to be proteins of average size. (The molecule of the botulinus toxin weighs 150,000 daltons, which is average for a protein.) As for plant toxins, they fall into several major chemical classes—alkaloids, glycosides, saponins. Toxins from snakes, spiders, lizards, and other animals tend to be small proteins (a molecular weight of less than 100,000 daltons.) And those animals that have evolved from a common ancestor of millions of years ago seem to have toxins that resemble one another even more. For instance, Dr. Schantz has found similarities among the chemical makeup of different species of blue-green algae. Also, snake toxins that act on one side of the nerve junction tend to be almost identical, whereas those that act on the other side of the junction tend to be identical, according to Dr. Rosenberg.

In fact, all snake poisons are proteins of similar chemical composition, reports Dr. Larry Rosen of Columbia University College of Physicians and Surgeons. In rare instances, animals that are not related may produce chemically related poisons. Tetrodotoxin, the poison of the puffer fish, is chemically identical to tarichotoxin, a poison found in the embryo of a California fresh-water salamander. "If you put the amino acid composition of scorpion toxin alongside the composition of snake toxin, you can hardly tell the difference," says Dr. D. D. Watt of Creighton University School of Medicine. And some toad, insect, and plant toxins are similar.

As for natural, nonbiological toxins, they are made of all the elements and in various combinations. Synthetic toxins run a wide gamut—industrial chemicals, pesticides, drugs, certain food additives.

Like and Unlike

Thus one can expect those poisons that are similar in makeup to have similar biological actions, and those that are different in makeup to have different biological actions. Still, there are some striking similarities among various kinds of poisons. Many, for example, act on the central nervous system. In addition, there are even closer similarities in action among some poisons of radically different chemical makeup. For instance, botulinus toxin and scorpion toxin both act on acetylcholine release. However, the botulinus toxin blocks the chemical, whereas the scorpion toxin releases it. Saxitoxin, the poison of one species of blue-green algae, and tetrodotoxin have identical actions. Different kinds of poisons can also produce similar symptoms. The symptoms of acute arsenical poisoning, for example—vomiting, diarrhea, abdominal pain—closely resemble those of cholera or of acute bacterial food poisoning.

Scientists don't understand these intriguing similarities. They would like to solve the mysteries. They would also like to answer a number of other questions about poisons. For instance, why do organisms make toxins in the first place? Dr. Halstead, who is one of the world's authorities on toxic marine animals, replies: "Biotoxins appear to serve as defensive or offensive mechanisms in food procurement. . . . This is an area of ecological research that has received little attention."

How many poisons are there in the world? Scientists haven't begun to count or discover all of them, especially in the ocean. In fact, Dr. Halstead estimates that no more than 1 per cent of all marine organisms have been explored by scientists. What are the chemical compositions of poisons? Although the formulas of synthetic compounds had to be known in order to make them, the compositions of only a handful of natural toxins have been worked out. For instance, the amino-acid sequences of only 20 to 30 protein toxins have been sequenced, Dr. Rosenberg estimates. And these are made of the smaller snake-protein molecules, not the larger protein molecules from microorganisms.

Finally, scientists would like to tap more poisons for good uses. Here again, the ocean holds vast potential.

Even with all these questions, though, scientists still

know a lot about the subject. And they are learning more every day. We'll now take a closer look at the various kinds of biological poisons—what organisms make them, where these organisms are found, what the poisons consist of, what they do in the body, the danger they pose to people today compared to yesterday, and what remains to be learned. Then comes a look at how these various poisons have been and continue to be used in beneficial ways. After that, we'll look at the incredible number of nonbiological chemicals both naturally present and artificially introduced into the environment. What uses do they provide? What dangers do they pose today compared to yesterday? Then comes the murky world of poisons used in suicides and murder —that is, their place in forensic medicine. Afterward we'll discuss the role that poisons have played and continue to play in warfare, in spite of worldwide controversy over such use.

Finally we'll look at what we can do to protect ourselves and our families from being accidentally poisoned, and what one should do in such a case. You'll probably be surprised by the number of poisonous substances stashed away in your garage, under your sink, and in your medicine cabinet, and by the number of poisonous plants that grow in your back yard or in a nearby forest. Who would ever suspect silver polish, aspirin, or fragrant lily of the valley?

2 · Toxins From Microbes

November 27, 1974, was like any other day for Gladys G. and Emily R., two widows living next door to each other in Griffin, Georgia. Because Thanksgiving was the next day, they shopped for some presents for their grandchildren. They had a leisurely lunch with another neighbor, Berthe B. That evening each ate a simple meal in her respective home. And the next day each went to her son's home for a Thanksgiving banquet. Neither Gladys nor Emily knew that the food they ate during these two days was going to change the course of their lives.

Right after Thanksgiving dinner, Gladys started to vomit. The next two days she complained of a sore throat, and her voice changed. Emily experienced similar symptoms, although they came on more slowly. On December 1, both women were in hospitals. By now their facial, tongue, and arm muscles were incredibly weak. The hospital staff drew samples of blood from them and examined the samples for toxins. Sure enough, they found what they feared: the botulinus toxin.

The major source of botulism—poisoning by botulinus toxin—is food. So a medical team set about investigating the food that Gladys and Emily had eaten during the previous several days. At first they suspected some home-canned green beans that Emily had put up. But when they found that Emily's son and his family had not gotten sick from eating the beans, they were sure that the beans were not the source. Then they learned from Berthe B. that the three ladies had shared a commercial can of beef stew for lunch on November 27. Gladys and Emily had each eaten half a cup. Berthe thought that the stew tasted sour and had eaten only a few spoonfuls. She did not get sick afterward. The team then located the discarded stew can and examined it for botulinus toxin. It was indeed the culprit.

Meanwhile, all the hospital's efforts could not save Gladys. She died the very day she was admitted. Antiserum (blood containing antibodies) to the toxin, however, helped save Emily's life.

Puny Organisms, Deadly Effects

It's hard to believe that such grave and lethal consequences of poisoning could have been caused by a minute organism that cannot be seen without a microscope. But the botulinus organism is not the only microbe to cause human poisoning. "Dozens of others have been identified," Dr. Gangarosa reports. And many of these small organisms make some of the world's most virulent poisons.

Why is this? Scientists aren't sure, Dr. Schantz admits. Perhaps it has something to do with the organisms' getting a head start in toxin production in the course of evolution. They are known to be among the most ancient life forms on earth. Fossils from some of them have been found in rocks dating back 3.4 billion years —an incredible time span. The earth was formed 4.5 billion years ago.

Of the several kinds of microbes that make toxins a danger to people, probably the best known type is bacteria. Bacteria are microscopic, one-celled organisms classified as Monera today, though they were once considered plants. They are present in soil and water and even in plants, animals, and people. Some are parasitic in that they depend on other living organisms for their nourishment. Many bacteria are harmless, if not actually helpful, to humans. These bacteria do not make toxins. Of the bacteria that harm people, about a third make toxins.

"These toxins," Dr. Gangarosa explains, "either cause disease directly or help the bacteria gain entry into the body or to further invade tissues. The disease is then due to the number of organisms present."

Those bacteria that produce toxins and that trigger disease in people include: *Clostridium botulinum*, the organism that causes botulism; *Clostridium tetani*, which causes tetanus; *Clostridium perfringens*, which makes gas gangrene, also stomach upset; *Corynebacterium diphtheriae*, which causes diphtheria; *Vibrio cholerae*, which triggers Asiatic cholera; *Streptococcus pyogenes*, which sets off tonsillitis and scarlet fever; *Pseudomonas aeruginosa* and other gram-negative bacteria, which can produce shock and death; *Staphylococcus* bacteria, which can harm the skin of newborns and elderly people and cause stomach upsets.

Another category of microbes that make toxins and that can harm people are the algae. These are primitive plants without true leaves, stems, or roots. But they

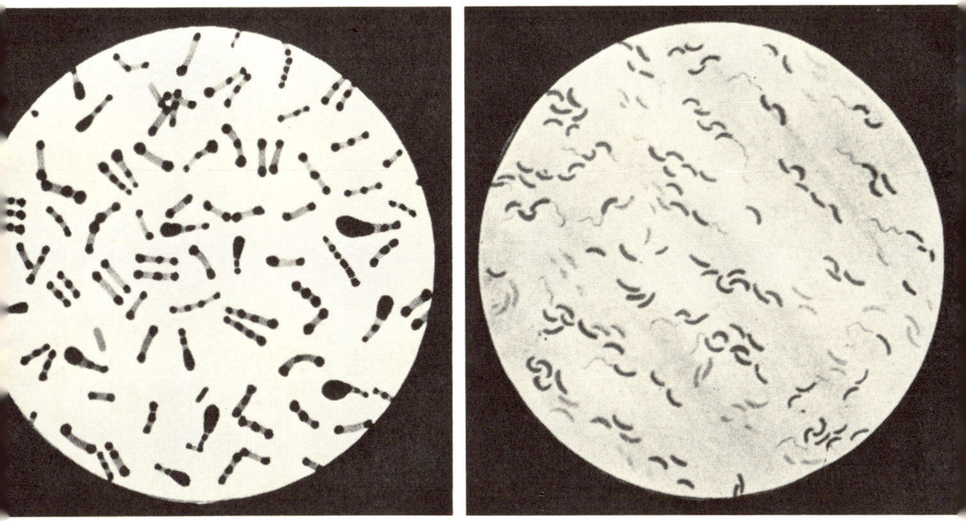

CENTER FOR DISEASE CONTROL, ATLANTA

About a third of the harmful species of bacteria make toxins, including those that cause diphtheria (Corynebacterium diphtheriae, *left) and those that induce cholera* (Vibrio cholerae, *right).*

always contain chlorophyll. Some are parasitic in their food requirements. Most, but not all, live in either fresh or ocean water. As a general rule, fresh-water algae are minute and can be distinguished from one another only with the help of a microscope. On the other hand, most marine algae, commonly called seaweeds, are visible to the naked eye and can be seen floating or cast ashore on the beach.

Many algae, like many bacteria, are harmless to people, or even useful. For instance, they are used to make agar for laboratory work, laxatives, and stiffening agents in ice cream and other foods. But then there are others that can seriously harm people. Prime examples are marine algae that cause red tides and some of the blue-green algae that grow in ponds and lakes.

Fungi, Good and Bad

Finally, another category of microbes that make toxins of danger to people are the microscopic types of fungi. Fungi used to be considered part of the plant kingdom, but lacking in chlorophyll. Now scientists have decided to place them in a kingdom all their own between plants and animals: Fungi. They are frequently parasitic in their food requirements. Like many bacteria and algae, fungi can do good things for people. For instance, they can impart a pleasant flavor to roquefort or camembert cheese. But other fungi can make toxins that can seriously hurt people.

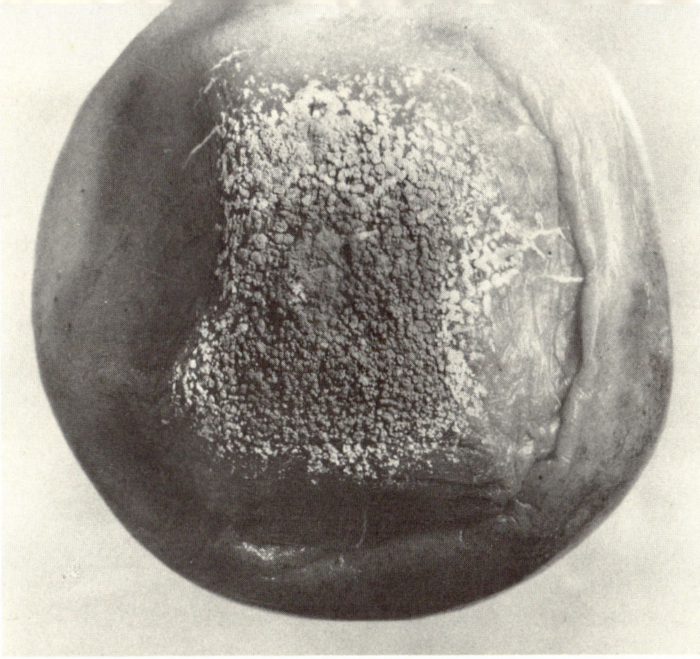

U. S. DEPARTMENT OF AGRICULTURE

Molds and other fungi are pretty much everywhere; this grapefruit has been destroyed by blue mold rot. More fungi that produce toxins are being recognized every year.

How many fungi make toxins? "Scientists don't know, but every year more are described," replies Dr. Libera Ajello, a fungus toxin authority at the HEW Center for Disease Control in Atlanta.

Food, obviously, is a major source of microbial toxins that endanger people. In fact, it is probably the most critical one, whether the toxins are made by bacteria, algae, or fungi. Of bacterial-caused food poisonings, about a third occur in restaurants, canning plants, and other food-service establishments. According to an article in a 1974 issue of *Food Technology*, the reasons are these: inadequate refrigeration; preparation of foods in advance; poor personal hygiene; inadequate cooking. For example, *Staphylococcus aurea* has gotten into salami after it was heat-processed. During the manufacture of iced confections on sticks, cooling water has sometimes been a source of contamination.

A good many of the bacteria-caused food poisonings occur at home. On August 24, 1975, for instance, some 26 persons who had attended a party in Gaithersburg, Maryland, were treated at hospitals for stomach upsets caused by staphylococcus bacteria. The bacteria had apparently been present in the chicken and rice that they all had eaten. The botulinus bacterium is most likely to slip into home-processed foods. About 90 per cent of all cases of botulism have come from them. That is why medical investigators first suspected that Gladys and Emily had been poisoned by home-canned green beans.

The botulinus bacterium is normally present in soils and streams. It exists in either an active form or in a dormant state known as a spore. The spores are incredibly resistant to heat, chemicals, and radiation. If they slip into carelessly prepared home-canned foods, they can grow there in the absence of air, resume their active form and give off toxin. When the canned food is opened, it may or may not give off a putrid odor advertising the toxin's presence. Such an odor was what saved Berthe's life.

As for bacteria-caused food poisoning of less certain origin, a prime example is that which many Americans get from eating foods in Mexico. For many years scientists weren't sure what bacterium was responsible. In the human intestine there are not only harmless *Escherichia coli* bacteria but also *E. coli* that make toxins. Dr. Gangarosa and his colleagues suspected that these might be causing food poisoning among Americans in Mexico and set up a study to find out.

The focus of their investigations was 133 American students on vacation in Mexico. The researchers took samples of the students' stools every other day for 18 days. They found that the day the students arrived, none of them carried the toxic *E. coli*, but the day that many of them got sick, this form did appear in the stools. So Dr. Gangarosa and his colleagues are convinced they have found the cause.

Red Water

Algae poison people through food by an even more elaborate route than bacteria do. Consider poisoning by those algae that form "red tides." Millions of one-celled algae of a particular kind congregate in the ocean. They give off a chemical that makes the ocean water look reddish or brown; hence the name. Why the algae suddenly reproduce in billions at one spot is not known. It appears to be due to a number of factors—nutrients, trace metals, and sewage runoffs in the ocean, water saltiness and temperature, winds, light. Once a tide forms, the algae excrete toxin in such large amounts that it contaminates fish and shellfish in the area. People can then be poisoned if they eat them.

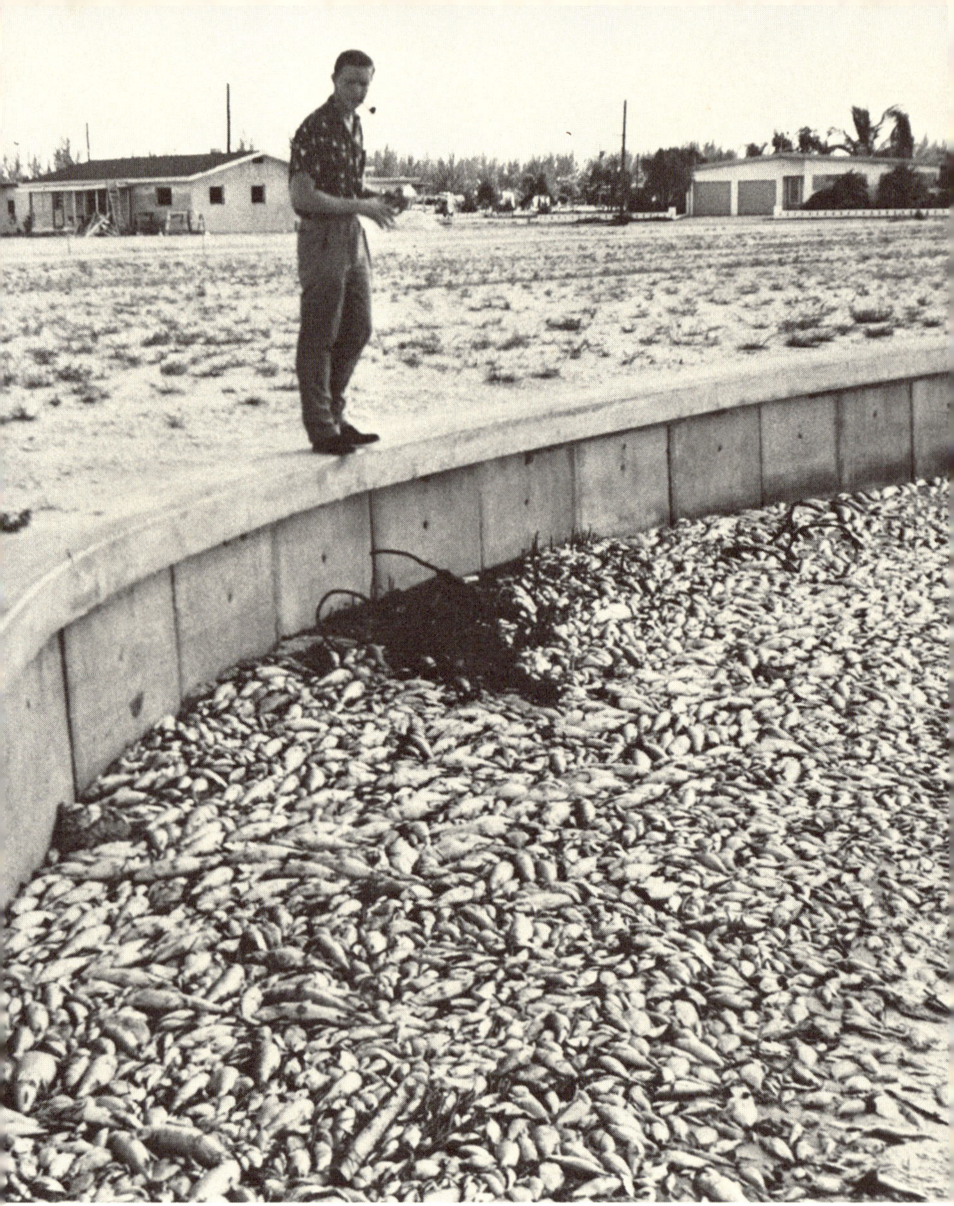

ST. PETERSBURG TIMES

Part of a large fish kill caused by "red tide" organisms, near Clearwater, Florida. The poison is produced by a microscopic one-celled alga, or water plant.

In the fall of 1972, for instance, the lower New England coast experienced its first red tide. Twenty-six people were poisoned by eating tide-contaminated shellfish. The Massachusetts shellfish industry closed down; public confidence was shaken. Even today the industry has returned to only 60 per cent of its pre-1972 level. And during the winter and spring of 1974, the west coast of Florida was ravaged by its twenty-fifth major red tide since 1844. A Sarasota boy almost died eating clams poisoned by the tide.

The toxins that poison shellfish, and in turn people, are made by various algae. The species that poisoned the New Englanders is called *Gonyaulax tamarensis.* Species that have poisoned Canadians are *Gonyaulax catenella* and *Gonyaulax excavata.* The species that almost killed the Florida youngster is *Gymnodinium breve. Gonyaulax catenella* threatens Californians.

As for toxic fungi in foods that pose a threat, they have been found growing in peanuts, corn, rice, cottonseed meal, oats, hay, barley, sorghum, and other staples. They invade whole or broken seeds and begin to consume the stored nutrients; that is when they make their toxins. Fungal toxin contamination is often irregular and localized. Outbreaks and incidences of toxins vary from year to year, commodity to commodity; and the contamination can even occur in just one part of a truckload.

Although food is the primary means by which microbial poisons harm people, toxins in water can too. For instance, blue-green algae have been suspected of irritating the stomachs and intestines of persons using a common water supply or swimming in ponds with water blooms, or accumulations of algae on the surface. The algae look like tiny flecks of dull green in a handful of pond water. A Bangladesh scientist reported in *Nature*, a British scientific journal, that he isolated a diarrhea toxin from the blue-green algae *Microcystis aeruginosa*. This alga is widely located in fresh water in many parts of the world. So the investigator concludes that the alga may be responsible for diarrhea epidemics and that drinking water containing the alga may threaten health.

Several unusual cases of bacterial poisoning through water contact were reported in the *Journal of the American Medical Association* by two physicians at the Ochsner Foundation Hospital in New Orleans. The bacterium at fault was *Vibrio parahaemolyticus*. This is a gram-negative bacterium (meaning that it doesn't retain a certain purple dye on staining) that lives in warm coastal waters during the summer and that contaminates fish and shellfish. So if people eat these foods, they are likely to get stomach upsets. In fact, the organism is the most common cause of diarrhea among the Japanese during the summer. However, *V. parahaemolyticus*' ability to poison people by invading their tissues in water was not suspected until the summer of 1971.

On June 27 of that year, 41-year-old Charles K. of

New Orleans was swimming in the Gulf of Mexico. He felt a sudden pain and noticed a puncture wound on his left foot. He thought that he had probably been stung by the spined fish called a stingray. For the subsequent 12 hours he felt no more than discomfort. Then he became feverish, perspired heavily, and vomited. He was admitted to the emergency room at the Ochsner Foundation Hospital and treated with drugs. He overcame the poisoning and survived. Three days later, bacterial cultures made from the wound on his foot revealed that the organism behind his poisoning was *V. parahaemolyticus.*

Then the following September 9, 60-year-old Raymond R. of New Orleans was also swimming in the Gulf of Mexico. After he came out of the water, he noticed that his right leg had been stung in a number of places. He didn't think much about it. But by the following afternoon he developed chills and fever, and vomited. Two days later he went to the emergency room at the Ochsner Foundation Hospital. By now his heart was beating irregularly, his stomach was bleeding, and his right leg was so infected that it had to be amputated. He died on September 15. Only after his death did doctors discover the cause; blood cultures taken from his blood grew *Vibrio parahaemolyticus.* They could only conclude that some animal must have stung Raymond while he was swimming in the Gulf, and the marine bacterium had entered the wound.

Botulism in Wounds

So it looked as if this bacterium's ability to poison people in the water was the result of its ability to get into tissues through a wound. Microbes' ability to poison people on land can also result from wounds. Botulism, for example, has been traditionally regarded as a food-borne illness. However, during 1971 and 1972, five cases of wound botulism were reported to the HEW Center for Disease Control in Atlanta. As with food-acquired botulism, the results are equally to be feared.

One of the victims was 15-year-old Mark P. of Sioux City, Iowa. He fell from a building and fractured his left leg and right ankle. Doctors repaired his fractures and gave him antibiotics and antitoxin against the tetanus toxin. *Clostridium tetani* has been well documented as a cause of wound infections. But they did not suspect that Mark may have been poisoned by another bacterium. His fractured leg and ankle became so infected that they had to be amputated. Mark then died. Too late the doctors discovered that *C. botulinum* had crept into his wounds.

And then there was 13-year-old Gary T. of Concord, Massachusetts, who injured his left thigh with a shotgun. He also received medical care, including tetanus antitoxin. But his wound became terribly infected. He too died, and the cause was discovered too late—deadly *C. botulinum.*

Still another victim was seven-year-old Jamie S. of Wilmington, Delaware. Jamie fractured his left forearm falling from a tree. He received surgical attention and antibiotics, but not tetanus antitoxin. He was also infected by *C. botulinum*. But he was luckier than Mark and Gary; he didn't die.

In reporting these results in the *New England Journal of Medicine*, CDC doctors Michael H. Merson and V. R. Dowell, Jr. wrote: "Although the number of cases is small, their epidemiological characteristics suggest that wound botulism occurs from spring through fall and affects predominantly young persons, especially males. The high prevalence in young males may reflect their greater participation in outdoor activities and exposure to soil."

As for the content of microbial toxins, many appear to be proteins with medium-sized or even smaller molecules. The chemical compositions of some of these proteins have been worked out. And investigators know enough to predict, in certain cases, those parts of toxins that are responsible for poisoning. For instance, the botulinus toxin fluoresces, or glows, in ultraviolet light. This in itself is not remarkable. All proteins fluoresce because they contain three amino acids of a distinctive quality. The amino acids are tryptophan, tyrosine, and phenylalanine. What is remarkable, however, is that whenever the fluorescence of the toxin is destroyed, its toxicity is too. So scientists at the Albert Einstein Medical Center in Philadelphia decided to knock one

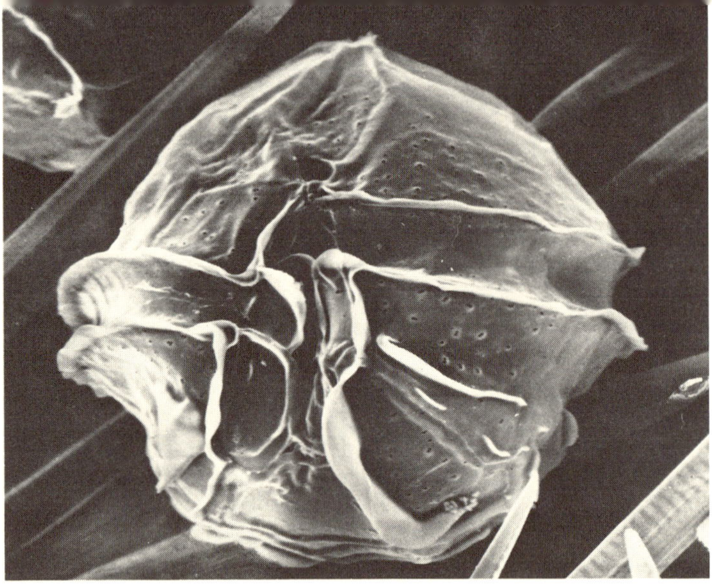

ALFRED LOEBLICH III AND LAUREL A. LOEBLICH, HARVARD UNIVERSITY

Beautiful but deadly—this is a red-tide organism, Gonyaulax catenella, *photographed with a scanning electron microscope and reproduced at a magnification of about 2000 times.*

of these amino acids, tryptophan, out of the toxin. As they anticipated, the toxin stopped glowing. So this amino acid at least is critical for the toxin's ability to poison. The other two may be crucial as well.

Not all microbial toxins are proteins, though. The chemistry of the toxins of a hundred or so fungi have been unraveled, and they vary widely. And then there is saxitoxin, which is made by the California red tide alga, *Gonyaulax catenella.* This poison's entire chemical composition and structure has been worked out by Dr. Schantz and chemists at Iowa State University. It's an incredibly small molecule, weighing about 400 daltons, and is one of the most toxic nonprotein substances known. It is a distant relative of nucleic acids, which are the genetic material of life. "It's a purine," Dr. Schantz says. "Purines are the building blocks of nucleic acids."

Symptoms and Deaths

The physiological actions of a number of microbial toxins are clear, especially those from bacteria. The botulinus toxin, for instance, first leads to vomiting and other gastrointestinal disturbances within 12 to 36 hours after being eaten. Weakness then develops, followed by dryness of the mouth and throat, with difficulty in swallowing. Indications of paralysis appear—double vision, drooping of the facial muscles, weakness in the tongue, neck, and extremities. Breathing becomes more and more difficult. Death is likely to occur three to six days after eating the toxin, largely because of inability to breathe. Recovery, for those who are fortunate, is prolonged, with considerable muscle weakness. The reason that the toxin is able to cause these various symptoms is that, as mentioned in Chapter 1, it goes for nerve-muscle junctions. The toxin inhibits the release of the nerve-transmitting chemical acetylcholine. Muscles cannot work as a result.

The tetanus toxin does just the opposite: it overstimulates nerves, which causes muscle spasms, especially in the jaws. The toxin binds chemically to the spot where one nerve connects (synapses) with another. This binding is essentially irreversible. Diphtheria toxin does not select only nerve tissue, as the botulinus and tetanus toxins do. Aside from making nerves and muscles degenerate, it can also damage the heart, pharynx, and kidneys. It binds irreversibly to cells within a few hours. The cells then lose their ability to make proteins. The victim may die suddenly from heart failure. If he survives, his muscles may be paralyzed.

Gram-negative bacteria can lead to blood clotting, shock, and even death if they get into the bloodstream. In 1975 Tennessee investigators found that there are chemical receptors on platelets—fragments from the bone marrow—that allow the toxin to bind to them. Such a finding, they said, is crucial because platelets are important in coagulating blood.

As for cholera toxin, it can trigger extensive diarrhea, vomiting, muscle cramps, dehydration, and collapse. If it is properly treated it is usually not fatal, and the victim recovers by the third to the sixth day after infection. However, complications such as pneumonia and serious skin infections can delay recovery. The action of cholera toxin at the cellular level has been extensively explored. Scientists now know that the symptoms of cholera poisoning, such as the diarrhea, are a result of the toxin's stimulating a certain intracellular messenger known as cyclic AMP. This stimulation then leads to an outflow of fluids from the cell. The toxin is able to stimulate cyclic AMP in the first place because it makes contact with specific chemical receptors as well as with several key enzymes in the cell. Local hormonal messengers—the prostaglandins—that operate between cells

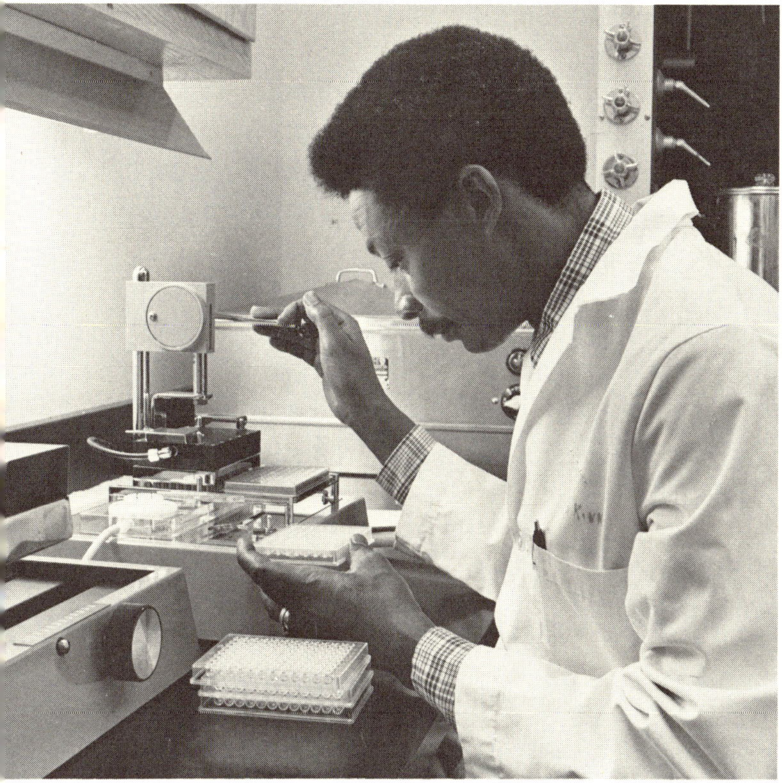

CENTER FOR DISEASE CONTROL, ATLANTA

Laboratory technician Fred McKinney makes an agglutination test to measure tetanus antitoxin levels in human blood. Tetanus toxin, unlike botulism toxin, overstimulates nerves and causes muscle spasms.

also help the toxin make contact with the victim cell.

Quite a bit is also known about the action of some algal poisons, notably those of the red tide. Eating shellfish that have been poisoned with them leads to symptoms only a few minutes afterward—numbness of the lips, tongue, and fingertips. Numbness of the legs, arms, and neck as well as muscle incoordination follow. The mental symptoms vary, but most victims remain conscious. As the illness progresses, breathing difficulty becomes more severe, and death can result from respiratory paralysis within two to 12 hours, depending on how much toxin was eaten. If one survives 24 hours after poisoning, the chances of recovery are good, and there appear to be no lasting effects from the poisoning. The amount of the chemical required to make people sick or to kill them varies considerably from one person to another.

A fish killed by the Florida red tide of 1974. The toxin interferes with normal functioning of muscles and in humans can kill by stopping the motions of breathing. JOAN AREHART-TREICHEL

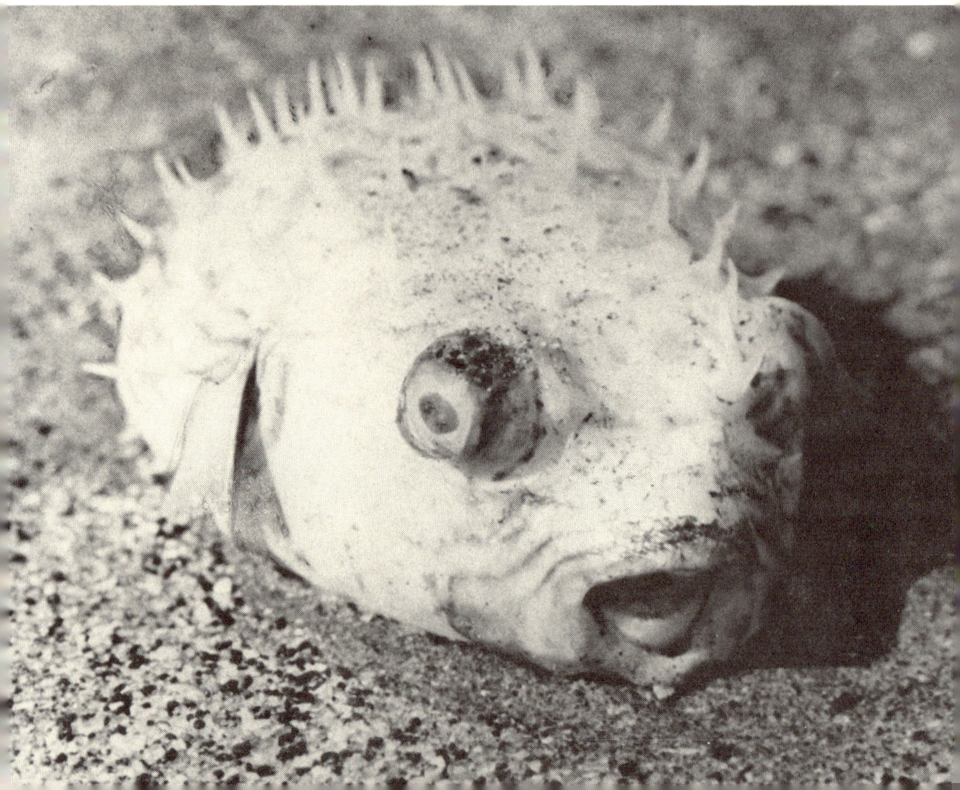

There is ample evidence that the Gonyaulax species exert their effects by blocking the current, created by potassium and sodium ions, that runs through nerves and muscle cells, and thereby suppressing the electrical activity necessary for these cells to function. The tingling and numbness that occur with the poisoning are probably the result of deranged sensory-nerve activity. As for *G. breve*, it has also been found to interfere with nerve conduction, as well as to break red blood cells, irritate the lungs, and damage the heart.

The actions of various fungal toxins have also been explored. Different organs may be affected, depending on which toxicant is doing the poisoning. Symptoms run from skin and eye irritations to upsets in hormones and nerves, liver damage, or hemorrhage. Even death may occur. For instance, a certain fungus, *Stachybotrys atra*, is often inhaled by Soviet farmers from dust and straw. As a result, they experience skin and upper respiratory tract infections. Bone and joint damage in Soviet adolescents has also been traced to fungi.

Getting on Top of the Problem

Thanks to scientific advances, mostly of the twentieth century, microbial poisons are not killing or seriously harming people to the extent that they once did. Vaccines have been developed against toxin-producing bacteria that cause tetanus, diphtheria, typhus, cholera, and staphylococcus infections. Antiserums as well as other sophisticated therapies are available for victims. For example, the death rate from botulism in the United States was 65 per cent from 1899 to 1949. Intensive aid to breathing and the elimination of the poison from the gastrointestinal tract, as well as the development of an antiserum helped reduce these deaths to 23 per cent between 1970 and 1973.

The development of better commercial food-processing techniques, such as pasteurization and putting nitrites and nitrates into cured meat products, has also dramatically reduced the number of harmful microbes in our food (though these chemicals are under strong suspicion of being harmful). Government surveillance helps too. For instance, the Food and Drug Administration uses a chemical assay on cross-country shipments of seafood to make sure that they do not contain red-tide toxins. Advanced transportation and storage systems, as well as the efforts of the FDA and the United States Department of Agriculture, have helped reduce chemicals from fungi in foods. As Dr. Benjamin J. Wilson asserts, "I don't think fungal toxins endanger Americans much today. The FDA and USDA are very much on top of the problem and watching shipments of grain, coffee, peanuts and other products all the time."

However, there are still many cases of microbial-toxin poisoning in the United States. The Center for Disease Control reported that from 1968 to 1972, 97,590 cases of foodborne diseases occurred. Two common causes were Staphylococcus and *C. perfringens*. Botulism has always been rare compared to other kinds of microbial food poisoning. But it is now increasing, Dr. Gangarosa reports, because more Americans are now canning their own foods than they were several years ago. In 1974, he says, there were 20 botulism outbreaks in the United States, twice as many as in 1973.

Increasing tourism has also exposed more Americans to toxicant poisoning through food and drinking water. Many countries do not attempt to make their food products as toxin-free as the United States does. Many also do not chemically purify drinking water. And even in the United States, with government surveillance, people continue to fall prey to red-tide toxins, especially when they eat fish and shellfish they have caught themselves. Dangerous fungi in foods continue to be a serious problem for peoples in developing countries. Surveys of foods in Africa, India, and southeast Asia routinely show large amounts of fungal toxins and cases of human poisoning.

So there is still a lot to do to reduce human poisonings from microbes. Fortunately scientists are making concerted efforts toward this goal. They are attempting to learn why red tides form, so that they can contain them. They are trying to predict red tides far in advance, so that people can prepare for them. For example, the National Aeronautics and Space Administration and the State of Florida are trying to make long-term predictions of Florida red tides. A satellite flies over the state, specifically the St. Petersburg coastal area, every 18 days and checks to detect any change in water color. At the time the satellite passes, a boat is sent to the same area to collect water samples from the tide. In that way satellite results can be compared with biological results.

Investigators are also purifying more and more of the microbial toxicants, then extracting those parts that can be used for vaccination without causing diseases. Such parts are known as "toxoids." But as Dr. Ruth S. Rappaport at Wyeth Laboratories pointed out in 1974, these toxoids sometimes revert to their harmful forms. So she and her team are exploring new methods of pulling the sting from them. Doctors are also trying to improve their therapies. For instance, they have found a drug, guanidine hydrochloride, which is thought to reverse the effect of the botulinus toxin at the nerve-muscle junction. They are attempting to find out precisely when antibiotics against toxin-producing bacteria prevent poisoning. And of course they will continue to unravel the chemistry of ever more of these poisons and explore their actions at the level of organ, tissue, cell, and even molecule.

3 · Danger in the Garden

It was a soft summer day in the country. Cattle were led from the village to the spring for water. While the cattle drank, they exposed the roots of a plant growing by the spring. The plant was water hemlock. This plant has delicate white flowers that resemble those of Queen Anne's lace. Soon after the cattle were led back to the village, eight boys and girls came to the spring to play. They noticed the roots of the water hemlock. Thinking they were tasty, they ate them.

Later the children returned to their homes. One of the girls complained to her mother that she hadn't gotten her fair share of roots. Little did she realize how lucky she had been. For about the same time, one of the boys who had stuffed himself on the roots, Jacob M., started to suffer from stomach pains. Then he fell to the floor and was seized by convulsions. Green froth oozed from his mouth; blood flowed from his ears. He cried for help, but his grief-stricken parents didn't know what to do to help him. He died.

This sounds like a fairy tale with an unhappy ending. Actually it is a true account from over 300 years ago in Europe. Jacob M. died from water hemlock poisoning. His companions who had eaten less of the plant than he also suffered symptoms of poisoning, but they survived. Water hemlock is one of the more poisonous plants of Europe and North America. And plant poisoning, especially among children, continues to occur.

How many of the 300,000 plant species throughout the world are poisonous? Probably several thousand. Seven hundred poisonous species have been identified in the United States alone. A handful of these plants, such as poison ivy, poison oak, and sumac are considered poisonous because they cause itching, inflammation, and blistering if one's skin comes into contact with them. The toxin in these plants is an oil related to lacquer. Sensitivity to poison ivy is acquired. Most people become sensitive through early contact in childhood, but become less affected as they age. Once sensitivity decreases, it rarely increases again.

Still other plants, such as ragweed and cocoa, contain chemicals that can produce allergic reactions if they are inhaled or eaten. Then there are plants that are considered poisonous because they can wound skin; examples are bramble bushes and desert catclaw. The plants that are poisonous to people in the real sense, however, are those that are toxic if one eats them. Many of these can seriously harm and even kill people.

Names and Dangers

Unfortunately a number of such plants are deceptively beautiful. Examples are lily of the valley, with its scented, drooping, bell-shaped blossoms, and monkshood, with its glistening green leaves and blue, white, or yellow flowers. Some of these plants have dangerously alluring names, such as foxglove, bleeding heart, or star-of-Bethlehem. Others, fortunately, have names that are more appropriate and that serve to alert people to their dangers, such as deadly nightshade or destroying angel. Plants that are poisonous if eaten can grow in woods, fields, lawns, gardens, or people's houses. Some are even foods commonly eaten, that become dangerous if taken in too large quantities.

Monkshood is one of the most dangerous plants that grows. Its roots have been mistaken for those of horseradish, and its greens have been used in salads with disastrous consequences. Mountain laurel, which bursts forth with pink blossoms in the Blue Ridge Mountains and other areas of the United States in the spring, is another native plant that is highly poisonous. Tea made from as little as two ounces of mountain laurel can kill a person. A troupe of goats once performed in a Philadelphia theater. The stage was decorated with mountain laurel. The goats munched the branches, and six of them died.

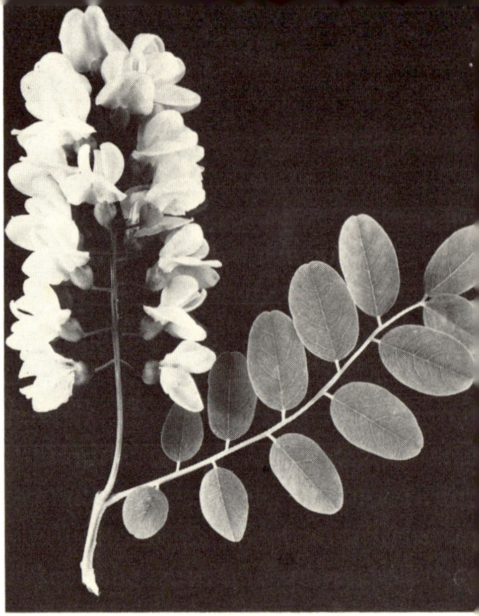

Two of the many plants that can poison if they are eaten. Top, black locust; bottom, belladonna, sometimes called deadly nightshade. U. S. DEPARTMENT OF AGRICULTURE

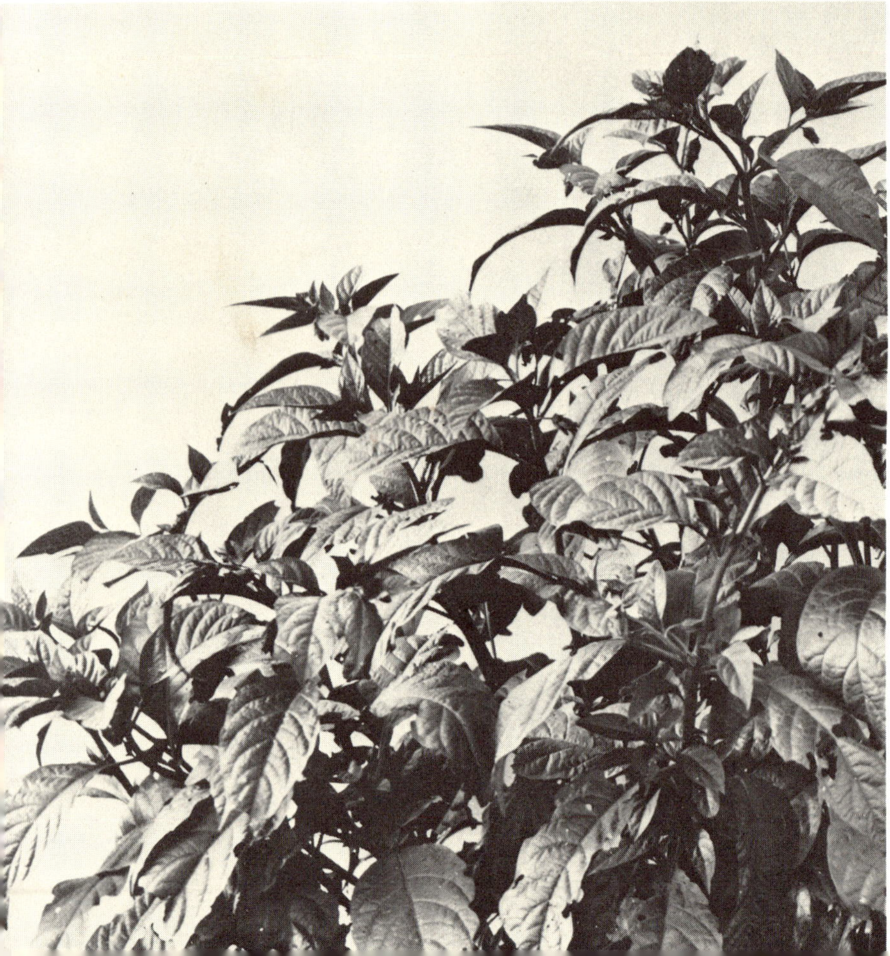

Then there is a weed three to nine feet tall, with lacy foliage, the poisonous hemlock. Fluid from it was undoubtedly used to kill Socrates. It is dangerous for anyone to use the hollow stalks of hemlock as telescopes or pea-shooters.

Deadly nightshade is another notorious poisoner that grows in natural surroundings. Its green stems contain luscious-looking black berries. If a child eats 20 to 30 of these berries, he can die. Lesser amounts do not kill, but produce delirium. The toxin they contain is belladonna —one of the poisons that witches used to "fly by broomstick" to sabbaths. The toxin's ability to create the sensation of flying has been confirmed by a twentieth-century scientist. He concocted a "flying" ointment according to an ancient witch recipe. The recipe included nightshade, baby's fat, soot, and several other ingredients. He and a colleague then drank the potion. They too "flew" all day.

Other poisonous plants found in woods and fields include beech, black cherry, black locust, buckeye, elderberry, jack-in-the pulpit, jimsonweed, Kentucky coffee tree, mistletoe, mulberry, oak, pokeweed, thorn apple, Virginia creeper. Back in 1887, 32 boys in a Brooklyn, New York, orphanage ate the bark of fence-posts made from the black locust tree. All were poisoned. Fortunately physicians were able to save their lives. And children have died from eating the white berries of the mistletoe.

Mushrooms and Garden Plants

Mushrooms are still another category of plantlike organisms that grow in nature and produce toxins. (Technically they're higher fungi.) Probably less than 10 per cent of mushrooms in the United States are dangerous, but that's still quite a few—about 90 species. Some of these poisons, like belladonna, give the victims hallucinations. A number can seriously poison and even kill.

The deadliest mushrooms belong to the genus Amanita. One of the most dangerous in Europe is *Amanita phalloides*. One of the most hazardous in the United States is *Amanita vera*, also known as destroying angel. "It's pure white, and one of the most beautiful mushrooms you have ever laid eyes on," asserts Dr. L. F. (Larry) Grand, an authority at North Carolina State University. "It is also one of the most toxic. One mushroom cap will kill a person. For a child or older person, it takes even less than that."

Of poisonous plants in lawns and gardens, one of the more virulent is the yew. This evergreen is used to landscape homes and has shiny red berries that attract children. Another notorious cultivated poisoner is foxglove. Its spiked purple or white flowers are, like those of a number of other poisonous plants, misleadingly seductive. According to European folklore, foxglove is a fairy

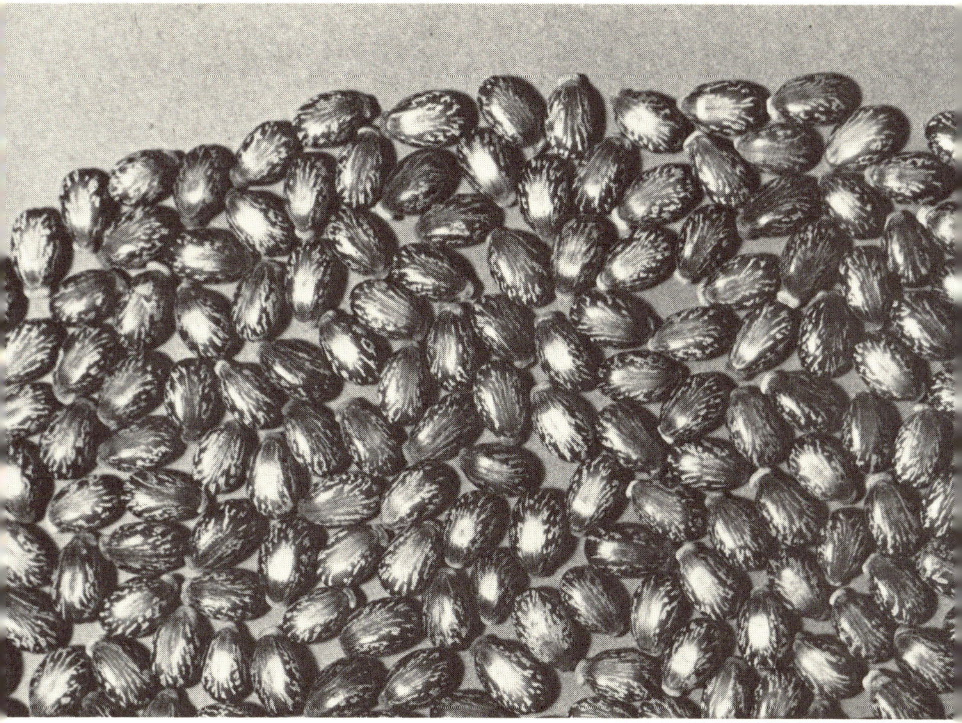

U. S. DEPARTMENT OF AGRICULTURE
Seeds of the castor oil plant, called castor beans, may attract children, who get them from this garden plant. They are deadly.

plant. Tiny elves are supposed to hide in its bell-shaped blossoms.

Berries from daphne, bulbs from star-of-Bethlehem, and flowers from the tiger lily are poisonous. All are cultivated plants. Castor beans, a mottled brown or tan in color, are produced by the castor-oil plant, used in landscaping. As few as three beans can kill a child. Rhododendron, a shrub with purple flowers, is a popular landscape plant whose leaves and flowers can kill. Zoo animals have died after being fed rhododendron leaves by visitors. Also, honey made by bees from the nectar of rhododendron flowers can poison people. And there is English ivy, which decks university walls and looks charmingly innocent blanketed with snow. It too is highly toxic if eaten.

Other cultivated plants that are poisonous if eaten include autumn crocus, azalea, bittersweet, bleeding heart, boxwood, cherry, chinaberry, clematis, daffodil, four-o'clock, horse chestnut, hyacinth, hydrangea, oleander, snow-on-the-mountain, sweet pea, tobacco, and wisteria.

Dumb cane and philodendron are two house plants that are poisonous if eaten. They irritate the mouth and throat and cause death unless prompt treatment is obtained. Poinsettia is still another house plant that is gravely toxic.

What, Potatoes?

Plant foods that people commonly eat and that contain natural toxins include the apple, banana, carrot, cauliflower, celery, lima beans, potato, rhubarb, tomato, and turnip. Fortunately these do not contain enough poison to hurt people unless they are consumed in unusually large amounts. For instance, apple seeds contain a virulent toxin. If a person eats several seeds, nothing will happen. But once a man who liked apple seeds saved them and ate a whole cupful at one sitting. He died. In still other cases, the reason that these plants do not poison people is that the toxic parts are usually not eaten. For example, the leaves of rhubarb contain far more poison than the stems, and people don't usually eat the leaves. However during World War I, the British government made an effort to conserve food. It recommended that people eat rhubarb leaves. Even though this recommendation was quickly retracted, many cases of severe poisoning and death occurred.

Toxins in plants vary widely. But there are several major categories. Alkaloids are one of the largest and most virulent. They are nitrogen-containing compounds. Belladonna, the poison of deadly nightshade, is an alkaloid. Aconite, the toxin of monkshood, and nicotine, the poison in tobacco, are too. Others include opium, from the poppy; strychnine, from the nux vomica tree in the West Indies and India; curare, from a South American vine; coniine, the toxin in poisonous hemlock. Potato sprouts, green potatoes, and spoiled potatoes contain a keenly toxic alkaloid. So do autumn crocus, hyacinth, larkspur, star-of-Bethlehem, thorn apple, and yew.

Plants aren't the only living organisms that make poisonous alkaloids. The puffer fish, for example, makes one that is similar to some of the plant alkaloids.

Glycosides are another group of potent plant poisons. Plants containing them include lily of the valley, horse chestnut, lima bean, almond. Digitalis and related poisons in foxglove are glycosides. Apple, cherry, plum, peach, and apricot trees and fruits contain the toxin hydrocyanic acid, a glycoside. One can take leaves from a wild cherry tree and put them in a jelly jar for a few minutes. On uncapping the jar, one gets the odor of bitter almonds, from hydrocyanic acid in the leaves.

Like poisonous alkaloids, toxic glycosides are made by some organisms other than plants. For instance, certain toads make ones that are similar in chemical structure to digitalis and other glycosides found in foxglove.

Saponins are a third category of plant chemicals that can seriously poison. They have almost the same composition as glycosides. English ivy contains a poisonous saponin. Alfalfa, beet, clover, lily, soybean, spinach, and yam do too. For a long time scientists thought that such saponins were plant products exclusively. Then in 1960 they found that two sea animals, the sea star and sea cucumber, make them as well.

Oxalates are still a fourth group of plant toxins that threaten people. They are soluble or insoluble salts of oxalic acid that are toxic in high concentrations. Jack-in-the-pulpit, rhubarb, and skunk cabbage contain them. Plant toxins can even be proteins. European mistletoe, for example, has been found to contain some protein toxins. As for mushroom toxins, they tend to be composed of amino acids, the building blocks of proteins.

What Happens to the Body

Just as plants can differ from or resemble each other in toxic composition, so can they differ from or resemble each other in physiological actions. Monkshood, for instance, acts rapidly and powerfully, producing nausea, slowing breathing, cooling the skin, and numbing the lips, mouth, and fingers. Deadly nightshade flushes dry skin, dilates pupils, dries the mouth, creates great mental excitement and delirium. Death results from breathing failure. Poisonous hemlock inflames the digestive tract, causes vomiting and diarrhea, slows breathing and induces convulsions. It also causes death by respiratory failure.

Yew leads to vomiting, diarrhea, delirium, convulsions, and a slowing of the heart until it stops. Tobacco decreases central nervous system activity. Death occurs when the muscles used in breathing are paralyzed. The nux vomica triggers such violent spasms that it contorts the body violently and distorts the face muscles into a hideous grin. Death is by asphyxiation.

Foxglove produces symptoms similar to those of yew. Apple seeds (in excessive amounts) and other foods containing hydrocyanic acid first stimulate the central nervous system, then depress it and usually lead to a rapid death. In some instances, however, poisoning occurs more slowly, characterized by dizziness, gasping for breath, convulsions, and coma.

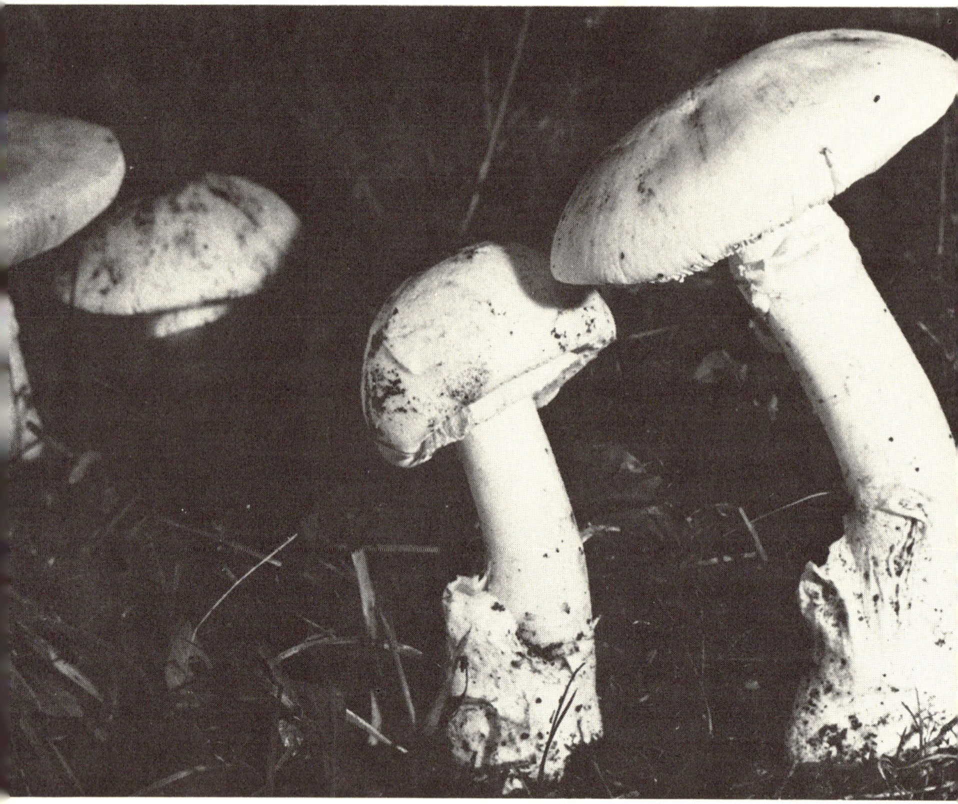

JOY SPURR

Amanita verna, *the destroying angel, is one of the deadly Amanita mushrooms.*

English ivy breaks down red blood cells. Jack-in-the-pulpit causes inflammation of the mouth and throat. Rhubarb upsets the balance of minerals in the blood and threatens the kidneys.

As for the Amanita mushrooms, the symptoms are abdominal pain, followed by cholera-like diarrhea, violent vomiting, and death. The mushrooms' toxins attack both liver and kidney cells. They can also harm the heart, central nervous system, and other organs.

There is reason to believe that plant toxins were a greater health hazard in times past than they are today. Ancient peoples had to learn by trial and error which berries, nuts, seeds, leaves, and roots were nutritious and not poisonous. They had to learn whether drying, soaking, pressing, leaching, and cooking could remove poisons from plants so that they were edible. Such learning went on for centuries. When Jamestown, Virginia, was being settled, for example, settlers mistook jimsonweed for a pot herb. Several deaths occurred before it was correctly labeled.

Today, on the other hand, people are able to eat foods that have been established over the centuries to be nontoxic, or at least when eaten in modest amounts. And foods commercially grown and marketed are overseen by governments for safety, which reduces poisoning risks.

The New Danger

Nonetheless, toxic plants still threaten people today, probably to a larger degree than most of us realize. Many areas of North America are still largely rural. Even though there is a constant migration to the cities, there is also a countermigration to the suburbs and small towns, where people once again have frequent contact with lawns, trees, woods, and fields. More and more families are camping and hiking in fields and forests that are unfamiliar to them. More and more are doing their own gardening or brewing exotic herb teas as part of the back-to-nature movement.

According to a 1966 book, *Daffodils Are Dangerous*, thousands of Americans receive medical treatment each year because they thoughtlessly or purposefully eat plants they shouldn't. Children are especially endangered, because they like to sample new things, and their bodies cannot dispose of poisons as well as adults' bodies can. An article in the October 1969 issue of *Science and Children* reported that plants are the sixth leading cause of poisoning among young children. A 1974 book, *Human Poisoning From Native and Cultivated Plants*, stated that 4.5 per cent of all poisonings in recent years have been due to plants. The number would be even higher if mushrooms were included.

How many Americans die from plant poisoning each year? It's hard to say. But annual deaths from poisonous mushrooms total 50 at least, according to a 1967 book, *Poisonous Plants and Fungi.*

To underscore the dangers that toxic plants pose to people today, let's look at some examples. People have died from eating green or sprouting potatoes. Scores of American children, like children in Europe 300 years ago, have died from eating water hemlock. Youngsters have been killed by eating daphne berries, star-of-Bethlehem bulbs, lily bulbs, poinsettia flowers, horse chestnuts, mistletoe berries. Wisteria produces poisonous seed pods that look enough like pea pods to confuse children. The toxicity of wisteria pods was first called to the attention of physicians in 1961. Almost immediately many unexplained illnesses in children were identified as wisteria poisoning.

In 1969, Karen S., a five-year-old from Washington, Indiana, drank water from a glass in which a bouquet of lily of the valley had been standing. Juice from the plant had oozed into the water and took the girl's life. In 1970 the Clayton B. family and Gary R. from Goshen, New Jersey, shared a stew containing wild mushrooms. They had gathered them earlier in a pine woods in Cape May County, in the southern part of the state. About nine hours after the meal, Clayton awoke with a severe stomach upset. Three hours later, Gary was sick also, as were Clayton's wife and two of his daughters. Gary, Clayton, Clayton's wife and daughters were admitted to the hospital. The attending physician was sure they had eaten the deadly *A. verna*. It turned out, however, that they had consumed *A. phalloides*, which scientists thought grew only in Europe.

In any event, Clayton suffered classical Amanita poisoning. His dehydration was successfully corrected, and four days after he had eaten the mushrooms, he was well enough to eat again. The next day, however, he became stuporous and hallucinated, then died. His older daughter died also. But his other daughter, his wife, and Gary survived.

"What It Looks Like" Is Not Enough

The basic problem with poisonous plants today, as yesterday, is that their appearance alone is not enough of a clue to recognition. There are other factors in addition that can determine whether a plant is poisonous. As was mentioned earlier, toxins may be distributed throughout a plant or concentrated in one or more of its parts. The amount of poison can vary with the season, weather or locale. A plant that is edible when young may be poisonous when it is fully grown. Some are poisonous when they are green—or else safe at that time. Adults as well as children are usually not well educated in the complex dangers of perilous plants. For instance, the precatory bean is made into jewelry in the tropics, then shipped to other countries. The bean is small, shiny and red, with a black spot on one end, and particularly appealing to small children. But what few adults or children realize is that one bean alone is enough to kill if it is eaten.

Even though more is known about toxic plants today than ever before, much remains to be discovered. Poisonous species need to be better defined. So do the conditions under which they are poisonous. Plant toxins need to be better characterized, and their actions in the body more carefully worked out. For example, scientists don't know much more about daphne than the ancient Greeks did. They have yet to identify its toxin. They don't know whether it is more poisonous in one season than in another, nor whether its virulence changes with location.

Still another question scientists would like to answer is why plant toxins are so poisonous. After all, plants also make alkaloids, glycosides, saponins, and proteins that are not harmful. Just as intriguing is the question of why plants create toxins in the first place. Is there some evolutionary advantage in the competition for survival? It's hard to say yes, because if a plant kills a predator, it is consumed in the process. Still, animals do learn to avoid poisonous plants; naturalists have observed this process in certain birds and mammals. So there might be some survival value for the species as a whole. On the other hand, at least some plant poisons may have developed accidentally in the course of evolution, providing neither an advantage nor a disadvantage in survival.

And, most critically, scientists want to find more antidotes to the poisons. For instance, there are not any sure-fire antitoxins for Amanita poisoning. One of the reasons that Gary B. survived *A. phalloides* poisoning was that he was given an experimental drug called thioctic acid. It had already been used to counter liver damage from heavy-metal poisoning, but there is no reason to think it can be relied on absolutely.

"In the next ten years, we should learn more about plant toxins," biochemist Trevor Robinson predicts, "especially about the means by which they inflict damage. The reason is that we now have a greater knowledge of molecular biology. For instance, we now know that the toxic proteins in castor beans interfere with nucleic acid synthesis. We couldn't discover this action until we first knew how nucleic acids are synthesized. The same thing is true with nerve toxins. We are only now learning how nerve growth and transmission work. Until we know how they work normally, we won't have a system to test toxins on."

4 · Animals With Venom

Becky and Josh J. were walking home from school. The hills were a tawny gold and smelled of Indian summer. One mile behind them, two miles to go. "Let's take the short cut," Josh said, "up Markham's Hill."

Shenandoah Valley children are taught to watch for poisonous snakes. But in October it was getting late for them, and Becky and Josh were preoccupied with crimson sugar maples and wood smoke in the air. Halfway up Markham's Hill they flushed a covey of quail. Their ears were filled with the chatter of squirrels and the plop of acorns to the ground.

Suddenly something grabbed Becky's ankle and wouldn't let go. It was a copperhead snake. Its fangs were tangled in her sock. So she had to twist her ankle to shake the snake loose. Josh then threw rocks at it, and it slithered off into the leaves. Pale and shaken, he raced ahead to tell the family.

Becky's father met her and tied a handkerchief around her leg below the knee. He used a pocket knife to slash the fang marks on her ankle. The pain was excruciating, but Becky didn't faint or scream. Her father swooped her up into his arms and carried her to the house. During the next several days she lay in her bed in a delirious state, racked with pain and fever. Finally, thanks to her family's care and her body's natural defenses, she survived.

The copperhead is not the only animal whose poison can kill people, or at least seriously endanger them. Far from it. Hundreds of poisonous animal species can be found throughout the world, and a number of them in the United States.

Some of the most formidable threats to people, and certainly the most notorious, are poisonous land snakes. Of 3000 snake species throughout the world, about 300 are poisonous. Of 120 species in the United States, 20 are poisonous.

The most virulent snakes in the world belong to the Elapidae family. All but one of the elapids live in Africa, Asia, or Australia and include tiger snakes, kraits, cobras, mambas, and black snakes. The only elapid that lives in North America is the coral snake.

The Viperidae are the second most toxic family of snakes. They include certain vipers of Africa and Asia, the puff adder and riverjack of Africa, and the asp of Europe. The third, somewhat less toxic family is the Crotalidae. It includes the rattlesnakes of North, Central, and South America, the fer-de-lance of Central and South America, the cottonmouth (water moccasin) of North America, and certain vipers of Asia.

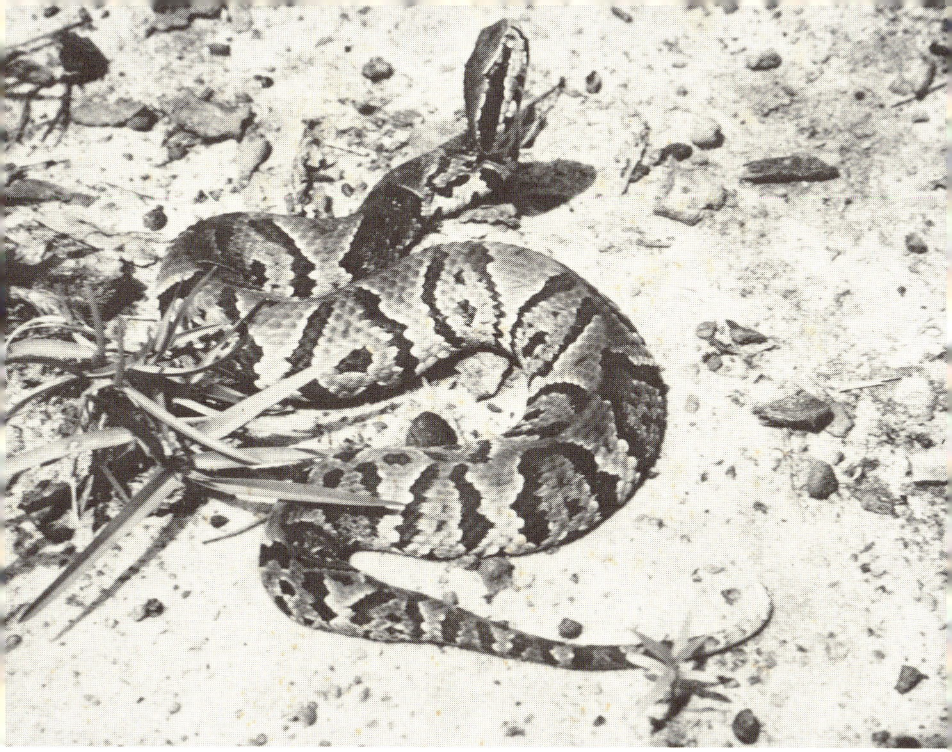

BOTH PICTURES, DR. SHERMAN A. MINTON

Two venomous snakes: top, a young cottonmouth (also called water moccasin) in typical threatening pose, photographed in Georgia; bottom, a coral snake, photographed in Costa Rica.

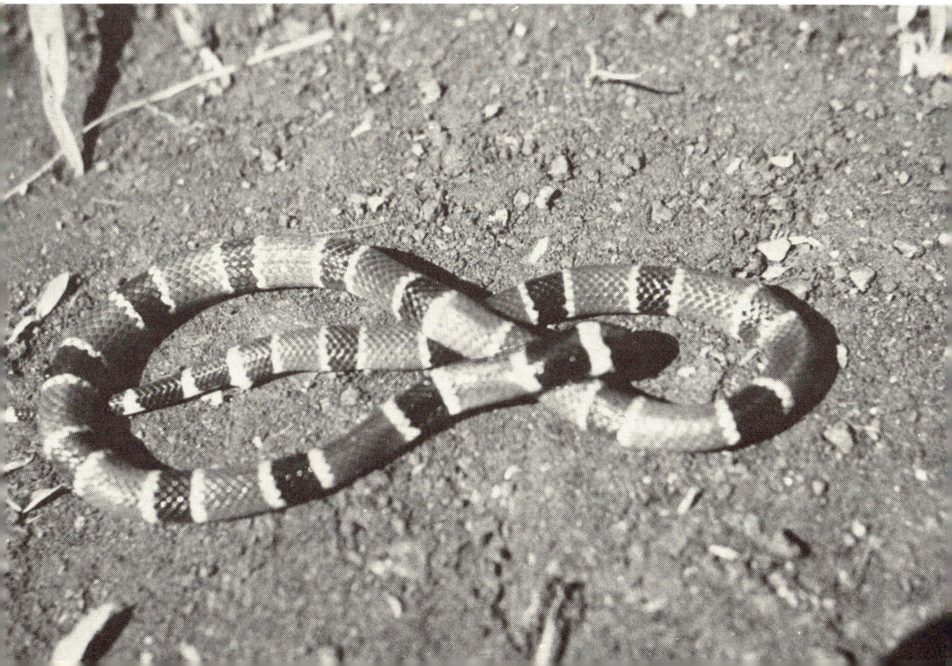

Pretty Danger and Rattling Danger

The coral snake is a deceptively alluring reptile. It has alternating rings of red, white and black on its body. The eastern coral snake, which lives in the deep South, has been described as the most beautiful of all North American snakes. The coral is a small animal of retiring habits and is seldom encountered by any camper or hiker. The western coral lives mostly in the deserts of western Arizona.

Rattlesnakes are found virtually everywhere in the United States, but become scarce from southern Maine to southern Minnesota. The prairie rattler's range extends into Canada along the borders of Washington and Montana. Rattlers will frequently give warning of their presence, but often not before they have taken time to coil and assume a defensive attitude. They are nervous by nature and will often strike upon little provocation if they feel they are cornered.

Copperheads are widely distributed from New England to Texas. Because of their retiring habits, they are apt to remain in comparatively large numbers in areas where the more conspicuous rattlers and cottonmouths have been eradicated. The copperhead lies quietly on old walls or in rock gardens, under haystacks or hedges. Its soft color blends with its surroundings, and it is easy to step on one before seeing it, as Becky did.

The cottonmouth lives as far west as Texas, north to southern Virginia and up the Mississippi as far as central Missouri. A large dark snake of menacing aspect, it is found in swamps and along turbid streams in the South. Some woods people say they can smell these snakes, although the typical individual certainly cannot. This is probably America's most aggressive toxic snake. It will not hesitate to strike if disturbed and it will bite under water.

Poisonous snakes and the harm they can inflict have both fascinated and worried humans for centuries. Consequently many legends have sprung up about them. For instance, there is a widely held belief in parts of the United States that rattlers actually hate people, especially those wearing blue, and will go out of their way to attack them. Scientists have not found any basis for this belief—nor for the one, mentioned in Chapter 1, that copperheads are especially likely to strike during the "dog days" of August. However, Israel Bonebreak, an old-timer in Pineville, Missouri, says that he has often seen harmless snakes attack people during the dog days.

Reptiles and Arthropods

Other reptiles whose poisons are of danger to people include the beaded lizard of Mexico and Central America and the Gila monster of the southwestern United States. They are both stout creatures reaching a length of nearly two feet. A caged Gila is usually sluggish and only too anxious to be left alone. But if exposed to the sun, it becomes surprisingly agile and dangerous. When it bites, it holds on with great tenacity, chewing the wound. The poison that flows into the mouth from glands in the lower jaw becomes diluted with saliva and gradually works its way in.

Scorpions and spiders are another group of land animals whose poisons are toxic. Scorpions that emit virulent poisons can be found in North America, South America, Africa, and Asia. All spiders, with the ex-

The Mexican beaded lizard Heloderma horridum, *one of the poisonous reptiles* DR. SHERMAN A. MINTON

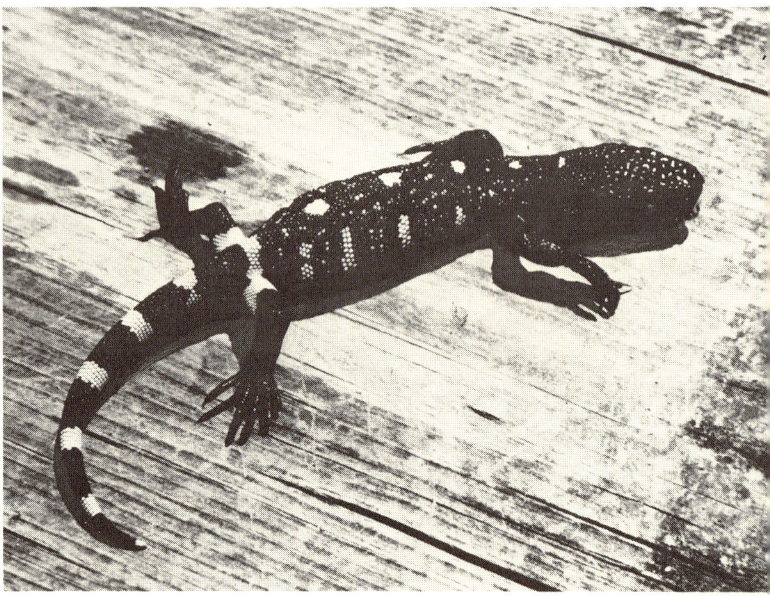

ception of two small groups, are venomous. Virulent spiders include the black widow spider, brown spider (also known as the brown recluse), jumping spider, trap door spider, banana spider, running spider, and others. One of the best-studied spider venoms is that of the black widow. It has been found to be six times more potent than the venom of the cobra and 15 times more potent than the venom of a prairie rattler, making it the most dangerous of all animal poisons. Fortunately the spider is small and is not able to inject as much venom as poisonous snakes do.

Other land arthropods besides scorpions and spiders that make toxins injurious to humans are fleas, bedbugs, ticks, mites, biting flies, mosquitoes, bees, and wasps. Bee and wasp stings can kill people who are unusually sensitive to their venoms.

The animals known as human beings make toxins too. As mentioned in Chapter 1 potent toxins can be found in human saliva, especially the saliva of children; they resemble rattlesnake poison. Whether they can actually kill another person through a bite is not known. Toxins have also been isolated from women's menstrual blood. If they are injected into rats, they kill the animals. What these toxins can do to another human remains to be seen.

However, people have been concerned about these toxins for centuries. European and American folklore says that menstruating women make hairdos droop and baked bread collapse. Menstruating women in some

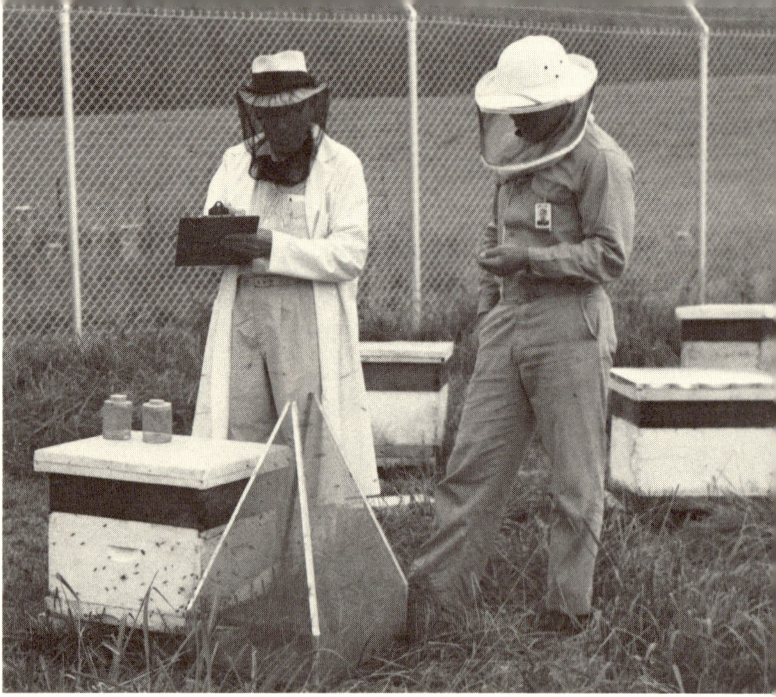

OAK RIDGE NATIONAL LABORATORY, ERDA

Two government scientists count irradiated bees in a behavior experiment, prudently wearing netting to prevent stings. The toxin of bees doesn't hurt most people but can sicken or even kill those who are sensitive to it.

areas of India are thought to be a source of pollution and are required to stay on the verandah until their periods have passed. Certain Pakistani women are prevented from praying while menstruating.

"I class the whole lot of these beliefs in the area of superstition," Dr. Virginia L. Ernester of the University of California wrote in the *Lancet*, a well known British medical magazine. Still, the myths may have some scientific basis. This writer has noticed that her hairdos really do fall during menstruation; perhaps this is tied up to a hormonal change during the menstrual period.

Sea Snakes and Other Marine Dangers

Poisonous marine animals are not nearly as well known as toxic land animals. But they constitute some of the world's most virulent creatures, and many of them can seriously injure, if not kill, humans. A prime example is the banded sea snake. It is the most poisonous snake in the world. A lethal dose of its venom, for dogs and monkeys, is 0.05 mg/kg (milligrams per kilogram of body weight). The lethal dose from the coral snake is 0.34, from the viper 2.0 and from the copperhead, 5.36.

There is a long-standing myth that one way to avoid being eaten by a shark is to wear a striped bathing suit. The reason is that sharks abhor anything in stripes because they think it is a striped sea snake. But is there anything to this idea? Dr. William Dunson, a Pennsylvania State University biologist, plans to find out. He will be serving for the second time as chief scientist aboard the research vessel *Alpha Helix*, a floating laboratory outfitted by the National Science Foundation and maintained by the Scripps Institution of Oceanography. On a previous trip to Australian waters, Dr. Dunson helped catch hundreds of poisonous sea snakes, often with bare hands. This time he'll dive off the Philippines, where banded sea snakes abound. He will try to catch sharks to see whether he can find any banded sea snakes in their stomachs. He will also experiment with baited and unbaited banded and plain

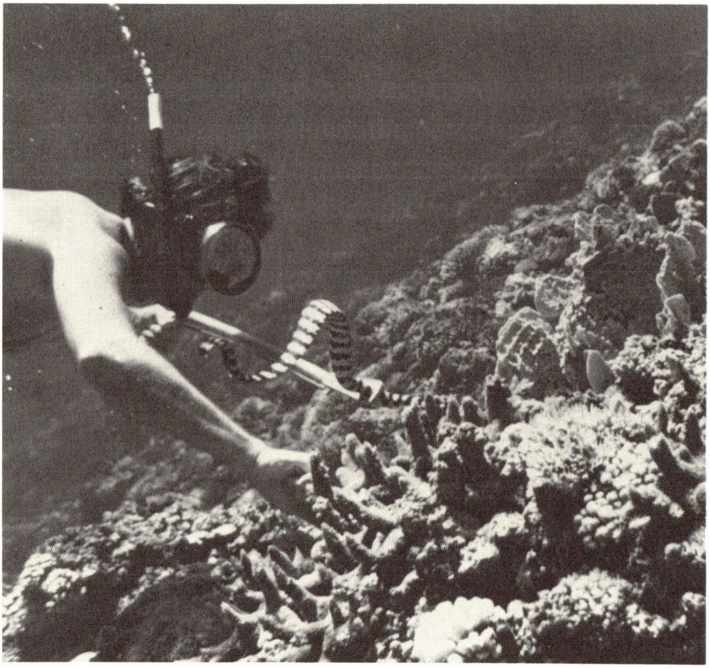

DR. WILLIAM DUNSON, PENNSYLVANIA STATE UNIVERSITY

Above, Dr. William Dunson examines the habitat of a banded sea snake he has caught; opposite, Dr. Dunson and an associate in the floating laboratory of the Alpha Helix *prepare a venomous sea snake for an experiment.*

poles to see whether sharks consistently avoid the banded variety, no matter what the bait.

Sea animals that can seriously poison people through their bites and stings include the stonefish, horn shark, dogfish, sea urchin, weever fish, Portuguese man-of-war, sea wasp (the latter two are jellyfish). Portuguese man-of-war stings have been described as resembling an electric shock. They can be moderate or severe, depend-

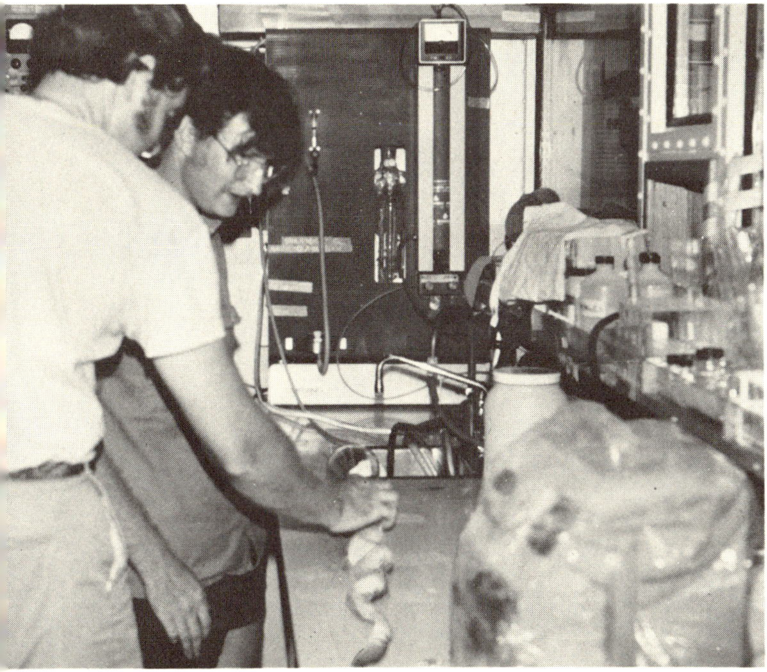

DR. SHERMAN A. MINTON

ing on the individual victim's reaction. The horn shark and dogfish can poison fishermen who brush against their spines while removing them from a fishing line. If sea urchin venom happens to squirt into the eye of anyone handling it, it can blind him. The weever fish's virulence has been known a long time. In the sixteenth century in Italy a widow pricked her finger with a weever spine and "through her negligence there followed gangerene and total mortification of the arm, and she finally perished miserably."

Then on July 24, 1955, a zoologist was skindiving near Naples, Italy. On the sea bottom he noticed a robust weever fish, partially buried in sand. The fish did not appear to be disturbed by the intrusion and allowed him to touch it. Suddenly it whipped out of the sand in a snakelike fashion and darted at the zoologist, first striking his face mask, then his jaw. He ex-

The Portuguese man-of-war injects its venom by means of nematocysts, stinging cells that are common to many types of jellyfish and related sea animals. When the "trigger" touches a prey animal it can cause the barbed filament to shoot out violently, breaking the prey's skin and injecting a toxin. Newer research has shown that nematocysts are more often set off by secretions from the prey animal than by a mechanical effect on the trigger, however. CHESAPEAKE BIOLOGICAL LABORATORY, UNIVERSITY OF MARYLAND

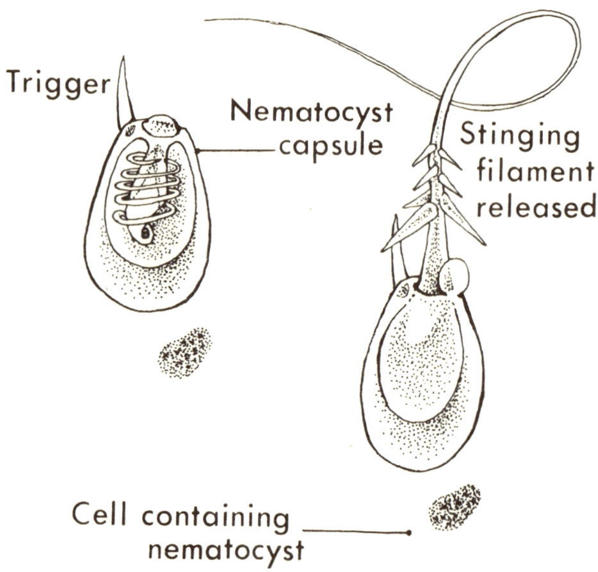

perienced such pain that he could hardly swim to shore. When he got there, his pain was so terrible that he begged people to shoot him. By then his jaw and chest had turned a hideous purple. He was rushed to a hospital. Thanks to good medical care and his body's defenses, he survived.

Still other sea animals that can poison people to a lesser degree through their bites and stings include the stingray, sea anenome, coral, sponge, and jellyfish (other than the Portuguese man-of-war and sea wasp). The stingray danger has been known for centuries. When Captain John Smith explored the Chesapeake Bay in 1608, he was stung by a stingray. In 1758, a Venezuelan wrote: "Children sometimes get stung voluntarily to get out of school or catechism. A clove of garlic introduced into the wound dissolves the blood coagulated by the venom and carries it away." Out of some 4000 species of sponges, about a dozen toxic ones have been identified.

A number of sea animals endanger humans if they are eaten. During spring and summer the ovaries of certain sea urchins are toxic if they are used as food. The horseshoe crab is also violently poisonous if it contains eggs, and can inflict death within 16 hours. The hagfish is also toxic if it is eaten. Turtles can become toxic without warning, and then are perilously poisonous if eaten. The consumption of shark, seal, walrus, and polar bear livers can likewise lead to violent illness. In the sixteenth century, for example, the Dutch navigator

William Barents was in search of a northeast passage to eastern Asia. He and his crew ran out of things to eat. Desperate for food, they then shot a polar bear. They ate it, including its liver, and became dangerously ill.

Probably the most mysterious marine animals that are toxic on being eaten are ciguatera fish. The phenomenon of ciguatera poisoning puzzles scientists. Many species have been implicated at one time or another, but snappers, groupers, moray eels, and surgeon fish are perhaps the most frequent bearers of this toxin. Also, the geographic incidence of ciguatera poisoning varies; an island group with no prior history of it may suddenly become toxic, then decline in toxicity. Or only one reef of an island may experience an outbreak. Since islanders have no easy way of knowing which fish are toxic, they usually throw one from each catch to a pet dog. If the dog shows no signs of poisoning, then the islanders eat the fish themselves and also give them to their children.

Still other sea animals whose poisons may possibly hurt people if eaten include sea stars and sea hares (a type of marine slug). Sea hares have had a reputation of being toxic since antiquity. One of the myths is that if a pregnant woman so much as looks at one, she will abort the fetus she carries.

Proteins and Symptoms

The vast majority of toxins made by poisonous animals appear to be proteins. Prime examples are those of snakes, the Gila monster, spiders, the Portuguese man-of-war, the sea wasp, and human saliva. And a number of these proteins are low-weight ones. As Dr. Sherman Minton, one of America's leading authorities on snake toxins, points out, these toxins "are quite different, for the most part from, say, the bacterial toxins like [those of] tetanus, botulism, and diphtheria. Those are much bigger molecules. They are also more complex than the toxins of mushrooms or other poisonous plants."

Snake toxins show striking similarities, suggesting a common evolutionary origin. As scientists have explored toxic animal proteins in recent years, they have learned that a number can be present in the venom from one animal. Snake venom appears to contain up to as many as 10 to 20 different kinds of molecules that participate in poisoning. Some appear to be toxins, whereas others seem to be enzymes that assist in the poisoning. Insect venoms also contain both toxins and companion enzymes. Sometimes the enzymes are even more virulent than the toxins per se. For instance, enzymes in the venom of the viper play more of a role in poisoning than toxins in the venom do. As Dr. D. D. Watt of Creighton University School of Medicine points out,

"We have found that whole scorpion venom contains not one or three or four toxins, but at least 25 different molecules, all with varying degrees of toxicity. All are low molecular weight proteins and closely related. We know the amino acid sequences for four of them." Spider and Gila monster venoms have also been found to contain enzymes that help poison.

Scientists are finding a few animal toxins that aren't proteins, however. The poison made by the sea cucumber—holothurin—has turned out to be a saponin. A toxic saponin has been isolated from the starfish. As for palytoxin, it acts like a poisonous plant glycoside, but it isn't a glycoside.

Poisonous land animals can produce a welter of reactions in the body, and in some instances, remarkably similar ones. Cobras, coral snakes, and other elapids, for instance, have been reported to cause drowsiness, thirst, nausea, paralysis of facial muscles, breathing distress, and circulatory collapse, leading to death within 48 hours. Their toxins attack the nerve-muscle junction and decrease the release of the nerve transmitter acetylcholine. Vipers, on the other hand, have been found to damage both the heart and the blood vessels in the lungs. And as for rattlesnakes, copperheads and, other crotalids, they trigger weakness, sweating, fainting, nausea, a decrease of red blood cells and blood platelets, changes in blood coagulation, in nerve-muscle transmission, and in the circulatory system. Death is usually from heart failure.

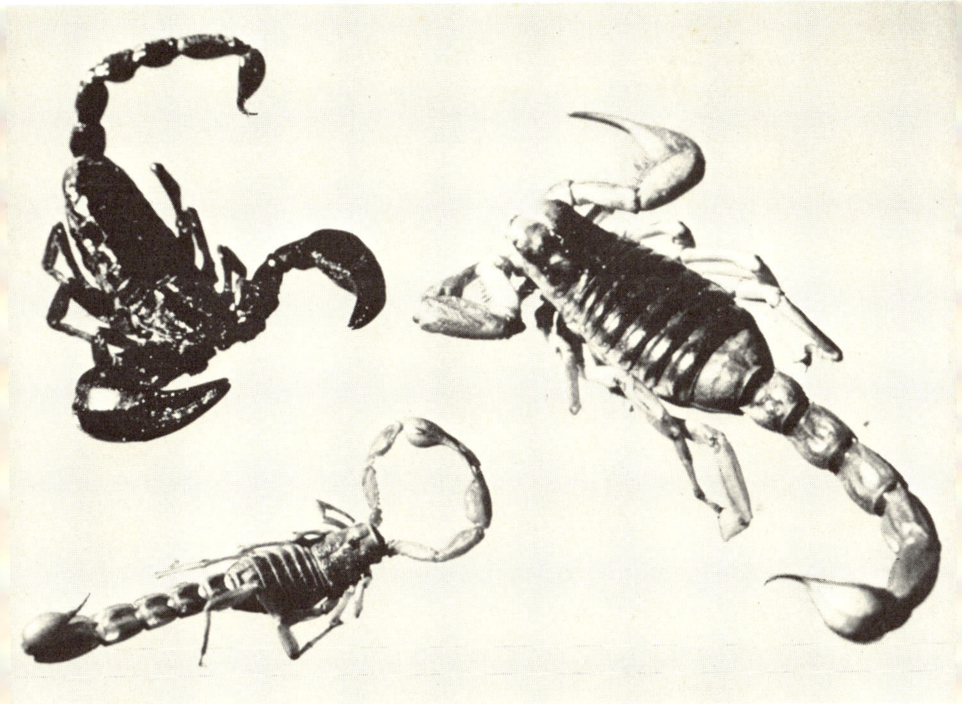

DR. DEAN D. WATT, CREIGHTON UNIVERSITY

Scorpion venom contains many different kinds of toxin. The black scorpion at upper left is from the Big Bend area of Texas; the other two, yellow and brown, are found in Arizona and the Southwest generally. Venom is injected by the sting at the end of the tail.

Scorpion stings lead to intense local pain, restlessness, hypersensitivity, spastic paralysis, respiratory failure, and collapse of the blood system. Scorpion toxin acts on nerves and increases their release of acetylcholine. This action is the opposite of that of the elapid snakes, which may explain why some of the symptoms of scorpion poisoning are the opposite of those for elapid poisoning. Death from scorpion bites, Dr. Watt says, is never predictable. Paralysis may go on for days, involving the heart and lungs. Or death may come within an hour after being stung.

A black widow spider bite can also produce muscle spasms. These spasms, Dr. L. L. Rubin of Rockefeller University has reported, may be explained by his discovery that black widow toxin attacks the nerve-muscle junction and increases the production of acetylcholine. As for the American bee, its sting can trigger high blood pressure in the lungs, followed by heart failure, Dr. S. J. Philips of Sinai Hospital in Detroit has found. The sting of the Russian bee, on the other hand, seems to produce a direct effect on the heart.

Poisonous sea animals can also damage the body in many ways. And some of these effects are also remarkably similar to each other or to effects produced by poisonous land animals. A sea snake bite, for example, leads to aches, pains, and stiffness of moving limbs. If death occurs, it is the result of respiratory failure. If a victim survives, it can take him five months to recover. Sea-snake venom appears to act mainly at the nerve-muscle junction, as does elapid snake venom.

A Portuguese man-of-war sting triggers pain in the lymph nodes, joints, and muscles and may be accompanied by headache, malaise, hysteria, chills, fever, vomiting, respiratory distress, and coma. In spite of these numerous effects, no deaths have ever been re-

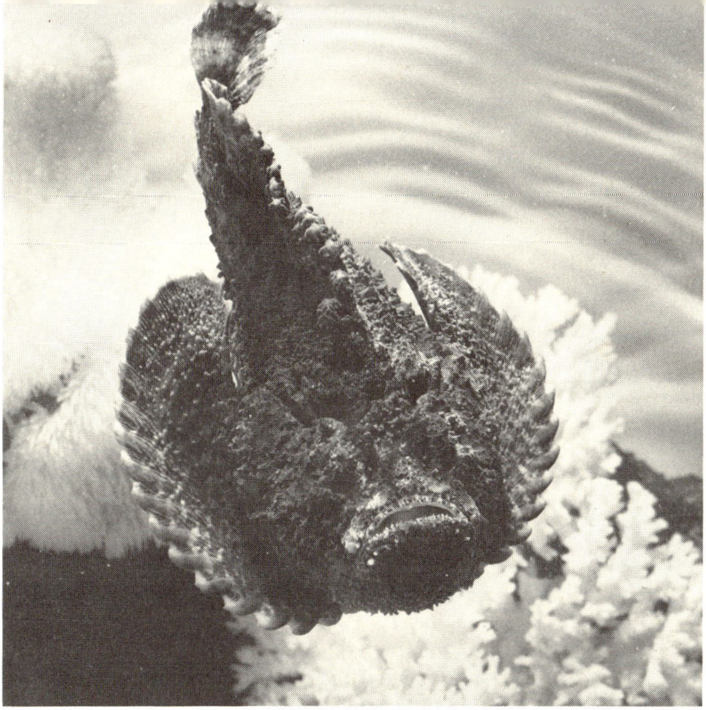

SCRIPPS INSTITUTION OF OCEANOGRAPHY

A wide variety of marine animals include poisonous members: such invertebrates as protozoans, mollusks, coelenterates (corals, jellyfish), sponges, king crabs; and such vertebrates as the stonefish shown here—one of the most toxic of all stinging fish. Other vertebrates include sea snakes, sharks, seals, and walruses, the livers of the last three being highly poisonous if eaten.

ported from man-of-war stings. Weever fish stings produce even more local pain than scorpion stings do. They also set off dizziness, nausea, collapse, and shock. Though the victim usually recovers, a sting can scar his tissue permanently. Fishermen who have had their hands stung by weever fish over the years often have deformed hands.

Jellyfish stings are rarely fatal, as mentioned earlier. But if death does occur, it can be in a matter of minutes.

Jellyfish venom is able to trigger high blood pressure and lead to acute heart failure. It may also lead to the accumulation of fluid in the lungs. Eating of ciguatera fish can lead to restlessness, salivation, sweating, diarrhea, abdominal distress, respiratory failure, and death. Ciguatera poison appears to inhibit a particular kind of enzyme found in muscles and other tissues.

A honeybee driving its sting, located at the end of its abdomen, into human skin. A bee sting can mean much more than a temporary pain to persons allergic to bee venom; deaths have resulted. U. S. DEPARTMENT OF AGRICULTURE

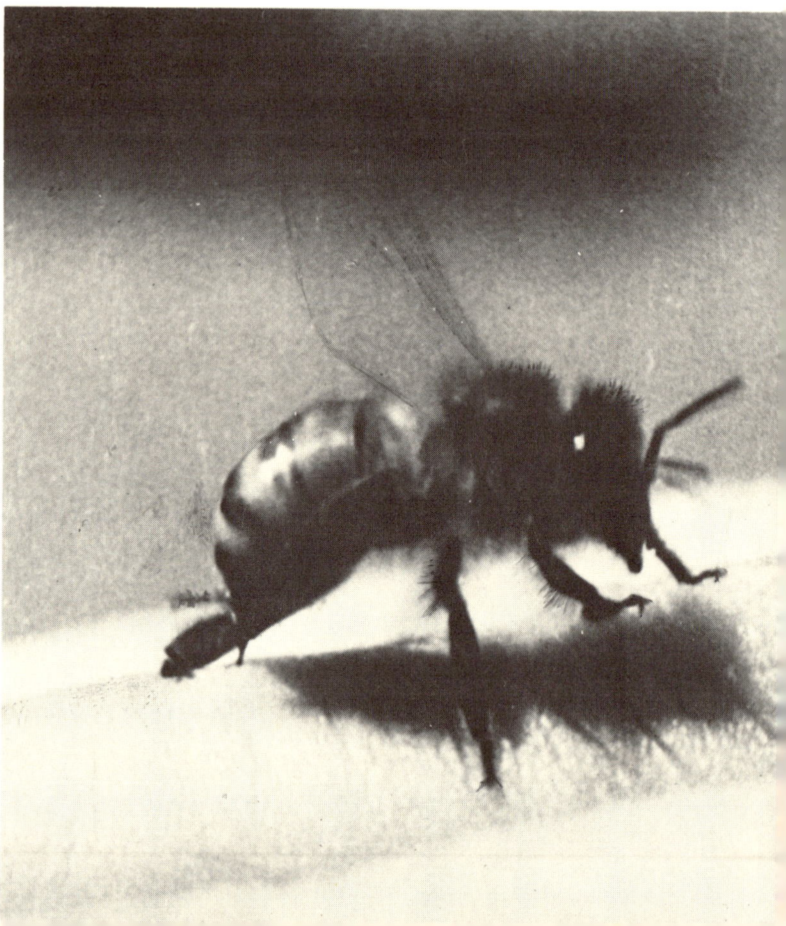

How Important Are Animal Poisonings?

Whether people encounter poisonous animals as much today as yesterday is hard to say. But the run-ins are still extensive, especially in rural and tropical areas. For instance, millions of people throughout the world are bitten or stung by poisonous arthropods each year. About one million are bitten by poisonous snakes; 8000 of these bites occur in the United States. An especially significant health problem in tropical countries is the consumption of poisonous fish.

And in a number of instances, such encounters lead to death or serious injury. Some 30,000 to 40,000 people die from snakebite throughout the world each year. Many more are seriously injured. In a study of 100 victims of rattlesnake bite, where antivenin was not used, 37 patients lost fingers, hands, toes, or feet. Fifty-eight experienced a loss in joint function. Deaths from bee stings are even more common than those from snake poisoning. They are three times more frequent than deaths from rattlesnake poisoning, Dr. Findlay Russell of the University of Southern California Medical Center reports.

Out of 70,000 scorpion stings in Mexico each year, 1200 result in death. Children are usually the victims. They are more apt to be bitten because they don't know that scorpions are poisonous. Also, the body mass of a child is small enough that the dose of venom can cripple, paralyze, or kill a child. Although there is a conflict over how deadly Gila monster bites are, they have been known to be fatal. Ciguatoxin rarely kills. But it does contribute heavily to public health and nutrition problems among people in the Carribean and South Pacific who depend on reef fish for food.

On many other occasions, however, confrontation with poisonous animals does not lead to serious consequences. Of those 8000 Americans bitten by toxic snakes each year, only 12 die. In New Guinea, where some of the most virulent snakes in the world can be found, 73 per cent of 193 snakebites didn't even result in poisoning. Of 824 poisonous snakebites in Malaysia, a good half of the victims escaped with slight or no poisoning. The reason that poisonous snakebites frequently don't lead to serious poisoning, Dr. H. Alistair Reid of the School of Tropical Medicine in Liverpool, England, explains, is that "snakebite in humans is fortunately a defensive reaction which rarely results in the injection of much venom. Thus, poisonous snakebite is not necessarily the same thing as snakebite poisoning."

Even though the venom of the black widow spider is extremely toxic, many people who are bitten by this creature recover. In 217 years, only 1300 bites have been recorded in the United States, and only 4 per cent have led to death. Nor do bites of other spiders usually lead to serious consequences. The reason is that the fangs of most spiders are too short or fragile to penetrate the skin. Nonetheless, at least 50 species of spiders have managed to bite Americans at some time or another and inflict damage. If a spider does manage to bite a victim, he should receive treatment by a physician.

Because of the widespread occurrence of animal poisoning among people as well as its often grave consequences, scientists want to learn a lot more about it. They would like to learn more about which animals in the world, especially in the ocean, can poison people. No more than 1 per cent of all marine organisms that make toxins have been explored, Dr. Halstead estimates. They would also like to understand better why animals make toxins, though there is reason to believe that in at least some cases they function in offensive and defensive actions. For instance, spiders use toxins to get food. And most of the ocean's venomous animals live in coral reefs, where they are especially vulnerable to being eaten.

Investigators want as well to elucidate the chemistry of more animal toxins. Says Dr. Minton, "We really don't know much about the venoms of a lot of snakes." Nor have the venoms of spiders been studied in detail. Fish toxins, Dr. Halstead says, are especially difficult to study because they are unstable, vary from one species to another and may even change within one species in the course of a year. The chemistry of ciguatoxin, spiny dogfish toxins, sea hare toxins, and sponge toxins is still a mystery. Investigators know little more about turtle toxins than they did a thousand years ago. Regarding the structure of palytoxin, Dr. Scheuer admits, "We are still working on the molecular structure and are not close to the answer." And how about the composition of human menstrual toxins? They too remain as a provocative challenge.

Still another area that biologists want to plumb further is how animal toxins exert their actions in the body. For instance, Dr. Watt now has reason to believe that scorpion and snake toxins poison cells by letting their disulfide bonds combine with the cells' membranes. Even more essential, clinical researchers want to step up therapies against animal poisons. Although antivenins are available against many snake venoms, this is not the case for poisons of spiders, the Portuguese man-of-war, the sea wasp, ciguatera fish, and numerous others. There is an antivenin against scorpion venom, but it isn't potent enough, Dr. Watt says.

If scientists are launching any ultimate attack against animal poisonings, it has to be in the area of prevention: the creation of vaccines. For instance, they have successfully vaccinated some Japanese islanders against cobra poisoning. A professional snake handler was successfully vaccinated against the tiger snake. Vaccines, of course, will be useful only among peoples who frequently encounter a particular poisonous animal.

5 · How Biotoxins Help People

In 1954 Dr. Leon Ciereszko, a chemist from the University of Oklahoma, snorkeled off Bermuda for marine animals that might contain unusual chemical compounds. During this search he noted a colonial marine invertebrate that looked like a carpet of little brown barrels set close together, and he was impressed by its ability to cling to rocks in brutal surf and to repair itself if injured. He subsequently found the organism in Bahaman and Jamaican waters as well. So in 1960 he decided that he wanted to learn more about the chemical composition of this tenacious, exotic animal. He collected a few clumps of it, then dried and stored it in a powder form.

By 1961 he and two students at the University of Oklahoma finally found time to look into the chemistry of the powder. While transferring it from one container to another for extraction purposes, they accidentally inhaled some. They promptly came down with sore throats and pains in their chests and shoulders. Dr.

Ciereszko went home to bed "with chills and shivers." That's when he suspected that the powder contained a potent toxin. And what a toxin it turned out to be! They had to get it down to a billionth of a gram so that it wouldn't kill laboratory animals. It eventually proved to be nothing less than palytoxin, which Dr. Scheuer and his colleagues found in Hawaiian waters the very same year.

This coincidental discovery of palytoxin set the stage for a new phase of research: seeing whether the chemical might be of some value to humans. During the early 1970s Dr. Pushkar Kaul, a pharmacologist at the University of Oklahoma, rose to the challenge. He conducted a series of experiments to determine the effects of palytoxin on various tissues, organs, and whole animals. The toxin adversely affected smooth and skeletal muscles, nerves, and blood vessels, he found. But its major action consisted of violently contracting the vessels that carry blood to the heart.

Poisonous Helps to Scientists

So Dr. Kaul is exploring the possibility of using palytoxin as a research tool to learn more about the physiology and pathology of the heart. For instance, it might be used to create angina pectoris in laboratory animals. Angina pectoris consists of a temporary inability of coronary arteries to supply sufficient blood to the heart muscle. It can lead to a heart attack and death. The only other way that researchers can trigger this ailment in laboratory animals at present is by surgical means. Researchers might also use palytoxin-induced angina in lab animals to explore the value of new drugs in reversing angina. Only short-acting drugs like nitroglycerin are now available, Dr. Kaul says, and longer-acting medicines are very much needed.

Palytoxin isn't the only biological toxin serving medical research. Rattlesnake venoms can be used to induce heart failure in laboratory animals and thus shed light on how the heart fails. Snake neurotoxins provide tools for studying how nerves synapse together. The venom of a huge poisonous toad from South America is a rich source of serotonin, a crucial nerve transmitter in the human brain and central nervous system.

Biological toxins are particularly of value to molecular biologists because they provide exquisitely sensitive probes into how cells work, Dr. J. R. Smythies of the University of Alabama Medical School points out. Neurobiologists at the Salk Institute are using a neurotoxin from the Indian cobra to study the action of acetylcholine at nerve synapses. Enzymes from toxic bacteria alter cell membranes so that more can be learned about them. Dr. E. Myles Glenn, a biologist at the Upjohn Company in Kalamazoo, Michigan, adds toad, spider, bee, and snake venom to blood platelets to make them release prostaglandins. He can then test various drugs on the platelets to see whether they inhibit prostaglandin release. Such inhibition would be helpful in treating certain diseases. The reason he uses venoms to make the platelets release prostaglandins, he says, is that they're cheap; one gram will last three years.

And then there is alpha-amanitin, an amatoxin made by the poisonous mushroom *Amanita phalloides*. It inhibits the one enzyme that makes RNA—the molecule that translates a gene's message into a protein. So it is useful for exploring how RNA is made in cells. At pres-

Though Amanita phalloides *is a deadly mushroom, it has its usefulness also, since its toxin helps research biologists to understand the manufacture of RNA in cells.* JOY SPURR

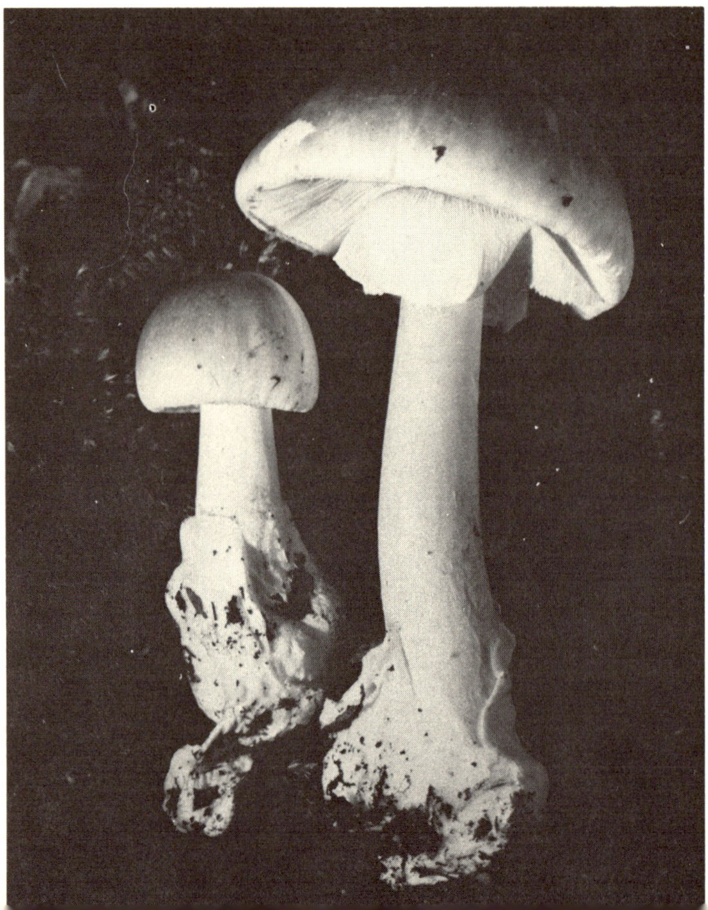

ent, though, the toxin is terribly expensive for researchers to use—$75 a gram. So Dr. Ray Holton of the University of Tennessee is trying to grow *A. phalloides* in the laboratory. In that way he could obtain a ready supply of the toxin for researchers.

Poisons as Useful Drugs

Biological toxins' greatest benefit to people, however, is probably not as research tools, but as drug materials. Biotoxins have long been used as medications, as mentioned earlier, and such use hasn't slackened in the twentieth century.

Foxglove, for instance, was used as a remedy in Britain as far back as the tenth century. In the sixteenth century its toxin was named "digitale," meaning "thimble." In the eighteenth century a doctor wrote an account of foxglove and of some of its medical uses. He was the first to recognize its value in reducing the action of the heart. Today it is called digitalis and is known to act directly on heart muscle. In the diseased heart it slows the rate of heartbeat, making the heart empty more nearly completely and thus increase its output of freshly oxygenated blood from the lungs. There are two digitalis drugs on the market in the United States today. Both are used for congestive heart failure.

Belladonna, the toxin of the deadly nightshade, was used in the sixteenth century by Italian women to enlarge the pupils of their eyes and to enhance their beauty. (Thus "belladonna," or "pretty woman.") The discovery of the toxin in it was made in the nineteenth century. It is atropine. This discovery set the stage for its use in medicine. Today belladonna is cultivated in the United States for drug purposes. Atropine is extracted and made into drugs for use in ophthalmology, specifically to dilate the pupil and paralyze the muscles of the eye; to diminish secretions from the respiratory tract; as a blood circulation stimulant, antispasmodic, and as an ingredient of liniments and ointments.

As for the glycoside toxins in lily of the valley, they were used as a drug to prevent apoplexy in the fifteenth century. Today the poisons are used to treat patients with heart disease. The toxin from the *Rauwolfia serpentina* plant was used in ancient India to relieve anxiety. Today it is used as a tranquilizer. Poisonous alkaloids from the periwinkle plant are used for treating migraine headaches and Hodgkin's disease. The hellebore plant toxin is used to treat heart disorders and to reduce high blood pressure. Opium, the toxin from the poppy plant, is used to relieve pain. Colchicine, the autumn crocus toxin, combats gout. Aspirin is a derivative of salicylic acid, a toxin in willow bark.

Modern pharmaceutical research promises to turn still more biological toxins into useful drugs. Cannabis, the toxin in the marijuana plant, helps control vomiting and nausea and stimulates the appetite in cancer patients, Harvard Medical School researchers reported in

1975. Dr. Sumner H. Burstein has found that cannabis suppresses the production of prostaglandins, just as aspirin does. So cannabis "may ease the suffering of asthmatics by restoring a balance in the prostaglandin level in the lungs' airway passages," he predicts.

A thrombin-like enzyme from the venom of the timber rattlesnake might prove useful in restoring natural heartbeats to heart attack victims, Dr. Bonilla has reported. Scorpion toxins might become muscle drugs. Bee and snake venom have been suggested for arthritis patients because they prevent inflammation in tissues around joints. However, Dr. Glenn and his colleagues at Upjohn have not been able to confirm this value. A number of plant saponins have antitumor activity, Drs. H. E. Wall and K. H. Davis, Jr., have reported.

If any biological toxins are going to become valuable drugs in the future, though, they are probably those in the oceans—simply because there are thousands there that have scarcely been tapped. For instance, scientists at the New York Aquarium have found that holothurin, the powerful toxin of the sea cucumber, may hold value for treating certain heart conditions. Holothurin has also been shown to possess anticancer properties in mice and a nerve-blocking action that could bring relief to amputees suffering from destroyed nerve ends. The poison extracted from the gland of a marine gastropod, taken from the coast of Norway, has proven to be a powerful muscle relaxant. Still another toxin, bonellin, discharged by a green worm of tropical and subtropical seas, has inhibited the development of the fertilized sea-urchin egg and has made the egg fall apart. This action suggests that bonellin might be a cancer-fighting agent. Red-tide toxins may prove useful as anesthetics, Dr. Schantz suggests.

Still other poisonous marine animals offer cloudy glimpses of medicinal use at this time—the sea snakes of the Pacific and Indian Oceans, certain viper fish, the jellyfish called the sea wasp.

The challenge in converting biological toxins into drugs has been, and continues to be, a matter of seeing that "they can be properly controlled and artfully used" by physicians, Dr. Stefano stresses. In brief, pharmaceutical researchers must make sure that the toxins can be given in doses that produce beneficial effects in a patient but do not poison him. And doctors must impress on patients the importance of not overdosing themselves with these powerful substances. For instance, digitalis is widely used by heart patients today. But they face an ongoing danger: the dose at which it is effective is extremely close to the one that poisons the body.

And then there are some biotoxins that will probably never be used as drugs, simply because they are just too poisonous even in tiny amounts. A prime example is palytoxin. Although this substance has combatted tumors in mice, Dr. Kaul fears that it will never be possible to use it as a drug for humans because of its overwhelming toxicity.

6 · Double-Edged Swords: Household and Garden Chemicals

During the summer of 1975, something bizarre and deeply disturbing struck the town of Hopewell, Virginia. Some 30 employees of Life Science Products Company felt nervous and anxious. They had trouble talking and experienced nervous tremors, loss of memory, and blurred vision. Some even became violent or talked of suicide. State health officials suspected that a chemical being made at the plant might have caused their illnesses and found that it was indeed true. The culprit was Kepone, a highly toxic pesticide that is widely used in the United States as an ant and roach poison. Kepone was found in the blood of the workers. It was even found to some extent in the blood of their wives and children.

The Hopewell drama is a tragic example of how nonbiological chemicals, whether natural elements or synthetic compounds, present a double-edged sword.

They hold great potential for good and have been largely created for good. But if people absorb them, they can do grave harm.

Indeed, it has always been this way. The early Egyptians, for instance, made use of crude arsenic, antimony, copper, lead, and other elements and experienced their toxic effects from time to time. The early Romans used lead goblets and plates routinely. Some historians believe that they suffered chronic lead poisoning as a result, and that this led to the downfall of the Roman Empire. However, people didn't really start using nonbiological chemicals extensively until the arrival of the Industrial Revolution, and such use has absolutely skyrocketed during the twentieth century with the vast expansion of the chemical industry. Consequently, nonbiological chemicals have presented toxic threats to people far more during the past two centuries than they ever have before in the history of human beings.

True, synthetic chemicals are woven into the fabric of modern society—energy, buildings, furniture, household products, pesticides, drugs, food additives, chemicals used in industrial production. Without them our lives would be far less comfortable, less pleasant, and in many instances even less healthful. On the other hand, we pay the price for their benefits. We are continually faced with excess exposure to them, resulting in the buildup of the chemicals in the body until they reach toxic levels. And there are too-hasty decisions to market some new chemicals without enough knowledge of how they might harm us.

The natural nonbiological and synthetic chemicals that benefit yet also threaten number hundreds of thousands. Some of them poison by being inhaled or absorbed through the skin or even by simply touching the skin. Many others, like most of the biological toxins, poison when they are eaten or drunk.

Killing in the Wrong Direction

Of the chemicals that poison by inhalation or skin absorption, the best known and some of the most toxic are pesticides. After all, pesticides, unlike most other chemical products, are designed to kill. So their toxicity for people is hardly surprising. There have been various instances of human pesticide poisoning, some of them dramatic. From 1965 to 1967 Dade County, Florida, reported 133 deaths among workers spraying fruit trees with organophosphate pesticides. In 1967 some 600 people became ill or died in Mexico from eating bread contaminated with the organophosphate parathion. In 1968 a father brought home a concentrated organophosphate to combat flies. He sprinkled it liberally around his house. He and two of his children were severely poisoned. Then in 1975 there was the Kepone tragedy.

Another group of chemicals that can poison through inhalation or skin absorption are the metals. Antimony, for example, can poison workers if they inhale its fumes. Gases too poison through inhalation and skin absorption. Firemen are often endangered by carbon monoxide in fires. In France more than a thousand miners were killed by carbon monoxide released after underground explosions. Miners are threatened by excess levels of carbon dioxide because it tends to accumulate in mines, being heavier than air. Although people are not likely to be severely poisoned by excess carbon dioxide in a room, there may still be enough to give them a feeling of malaise. Hydrogen cyanide is a gas widely used in industry, especially in making plastics. If absorbed into the body, it too can kill.

Still other, less known chemicals can poison people through inhalation or entering the skin. On May 26, 1971, waste-oil sludge was sprayed on a riding arena in Missouri to control dust. Three days later sparrows living near the arena died. Several weeks later hundreds of birds, 48 horses, numerous rodents, and several cats and dogs also succumbed. Although the several children and adults using the arena didn't die, they were moderately poisoned. So the arena soil was analyzed for a noxious chemical. One was indeed found. It was a chlorinated dibenzodioxin. This class of compounds is found in products like waste-oil sludge. Some of them are highly toxic.

The deadly radioactive elements also poison by being taken into the lungs or skin. Persons who work in nuclear energy plants or in diagnosing and treating patients with radiation are more likely to encounter such elements than is the general population.

One of the major chemicals that can poison by touch-

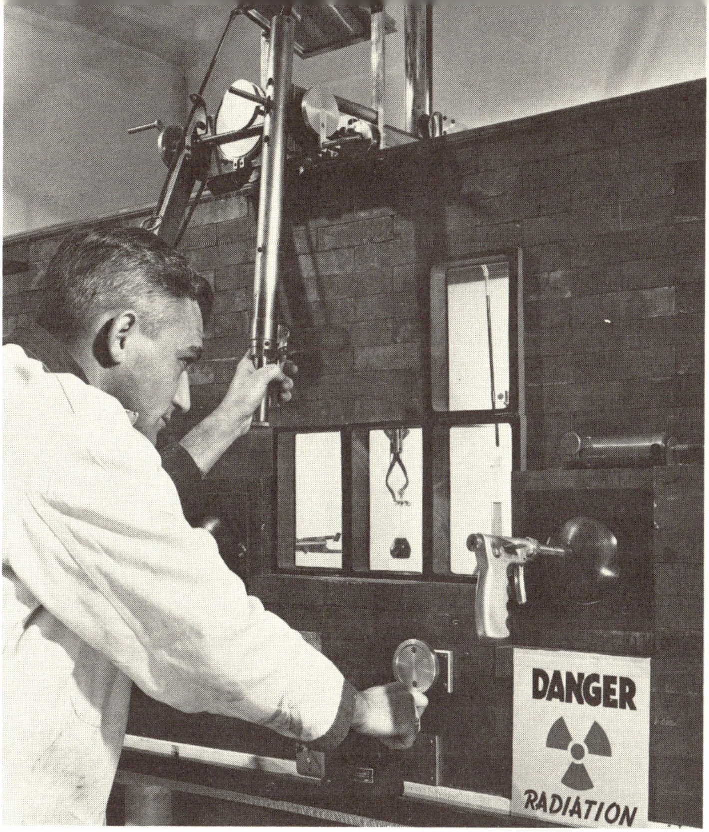

BROOKHAVEN NATIONAL LABORATORY

Radioactive elements can poison research and medical workers unless they are extremely careful with them. This physicist is using remote-control manipulators to handle a dangerous flask in a radioactively "hot" area.

ing the skin is carbolic acid, a common disinfectant used at home and in the hospitals. Ammonia water, used for cleaning and bleaching at home, gives off fumes that can poison the skin and cause choking and gasping if strongly inhaled. Sulfuric acid, hydrochloric acid, caustic soda, caustic potash, zinc chloride, and silver nitrate are still other industrial and household products that can poison through the skin.

Poisons by Mouth

As for chemicals that poison by the stomach route, some of the best examples are metals. From 1953 to 1960, over a hundred Japanese were poisoned after eating fish and shellfish contaminated by mercury in Japan's Minimata Bay. Antimony is used in prescription cough syrups and other drugs. If the very young or very old consume too much, they can be poisoned. Iodine, used as an antiseptic, can seriously poison children if they drink it. Eating lead paint can do likewise. Making vitamins chewable and tasty for youngsters was a good idea, on one hand; on the other, it encourages them to eat too many, and there is enough iron in some vitamin bottles to kill a child. As mentioned earlier, some persons living in Alpine communities eat arsenic as a love potion, and to make breathing easier. Although some of them build up a tolerance to this mineral, others become sick from it eventually.

Drugs are another major category of chemicals that can poison when they are taken in accidentally. Aspirin is a leading cause of poisoning among children, barbiturates among adults. Narcotics addicts often die from accidentally overdosing themselves on morphine and heroin. A number of household products can also poison those who accidentally drink or eat them—rat poison, ammonia water, turpentine, furniture polish, oxalic acid, chloroform, alcohol, ether, and others. Children have died from eating mothballs, thinking they were candies. An amateur photographer narrowly missed death when he mistook a potassium cyanide solution (used for treating negatives) for lemonade.

Nor are people immune from accidental ingestion of toxic chemicals in food. PCBs (polychlorinated biphenyls) are chemicals used in the manufacture of plastics, paints, inks, and other products. They are dumped into waterways after use and occasionally end up in fish. On August 8, 1975, for example, state officials warned consumers not to eat bass from the Hudson River in New York or salmon from Lake Ontario because researchers had found that the fish contained dangerously high levels of PCBs. Food additives can also poison from time to time. Once 150 children were poisoned when they ate popcorn colored with a particular dye.

Molecules of Poisons

The chemistry of nonbiological poisons runs the entire chemical spectrum. Whereas the biological toxins are comprised mostly of six elements—carbon, hydrogen, nitrogen, oxygen, sulfur, and phosphorus—nonbiological poisons are composed of every conceivable element and in every conceivable combination. Even those compounds that are made mostly of the same elements that occur in biological toxins differ markedly in their elemental composition. For instance, the pesticide DDT contains carbon, hydrogen, and chlorine. Aspirin is made of carbon, hydrogen, and oxygen. Hydrogen cyanide comprises hydrogen, carbon, and nitrogen.

Nonetheless, the compositions and structures of the nonbiological poisons are precisely what determine their toxicity, as is the case with biological toxins. For instance, the organophosphate pesticides, despite their diversity in structure, all owe their toxicity to the action of a central phosphorus atom. The key feature of the carbamate insecticides, on the other hand, is a bulky side chain, or branched chain of atoms attached to the central part of the molecule.

Consequently the nonbiological chemicals can hurt the body in many ways. The chlorinated hydrocarbons, for instance, which include DDT, aldrin, dieldrin, Kepone, PCBs, chlordane, and heptachlor, attack peripheral nerves or ganglia in the central nervous system. Their precise site of attack is still unknown. Although they generally do not cause acute poisoning, such as trembling, convulsions, paralysis of the muscles, and coma, unless when they are absorbed in massive doses, they may cause subacute poisoning, such as nausea, vomiting, and diarrhea. They may also do serious damage to the nervous system if they are absorbed into the body in small amounts over a period of time, as the Kepone tragedy and a study of pesticide workers have revealed. In this study, pesticide workers were found

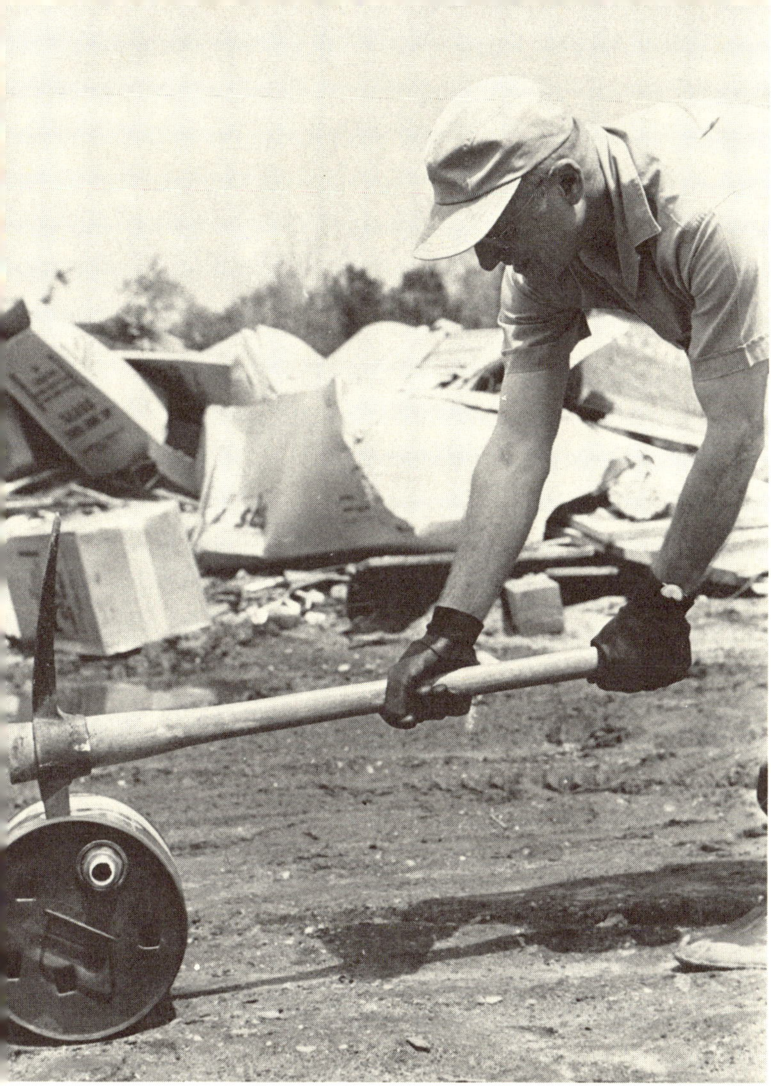

U. S. DEPARTMENT OF AGRICULTURE

Nonbiological chemicals such as pesticides, when used at all, must be applied according to strict guidelines, and empty containers for them should be punctured so they will not be used again (except in the case of pressure spray cans). Such containers should then be buried. Measures like these help reduce the danger of spreading such two-edged poisonous chemicals.

to experience drowsiness, forgetfulness, fatigue, visual difficulties, sleep disruptions and brain wave disturbances.

Parathion, Malathion, and other organophosphates, on the other hand, are always dangerous for humans. They inhibit the enzyme cholinesterase, which is vital for proper nerve function. As a result the nerve chemical acetylcholine is not removed from the nerve synapse. This obstruction can lead to nausea, salivation, giddiness, convulsions, and coma. For instance, children once rolled in a field that had just been sprayed with an organophosphate and experienced these symptoms of poisoning.

As for isolan, dimetilan, and other carbamates, the third major category of pesticides in use today, they too are always dangerous. Like the organophosphates, they inhibit cholinesterase, leading to violent convulsions and other neuromuscular disturbances.

Gases poison by various methods too. Carbon monoxide, for example, attaches itself to hemoglobin, so that it can no longer carry out its function of transporting oxygen. The shortage of oxygen then affects the central nervous system, leading to stupor, giddiness, and weakness. The victim panics and tries to escape, and in so doing uses up his last reserves of oxygen. When he is found he has an eerie rosy glow and is in a coma, if not dead. Hydrogen cyanide, on the other hand, doesn't interfere with the transport of oxygen. It blocks enzymes that cells need in order to breathe. So whereas the blood may be rich in oxygen, cells die from lack of it. Symptoms include difficulty in breathing, collapse, loss of consciousness, convulsions, and cessation of breathing, resulting of course in death.

Radioactive elements do their poisoning in a unique way—by detaching electrons from themselves. The electrons then strike cells and damage them, especially their nuclei. It is the repetition of such bombardment that is especially dangerous. The effects of radiation poisoning were well demonstrated after American planes dropped atomic bombs in Japan in 1945. Victims experienced prostration, high fever, vomiting, and diarrhea. Many also suffered serious damage to their nervous systems and died.

Carbolic acid and related acids exert a powerful corrosive action that kills skin tissues with which they come into contact. The top part of the skin then becomes whitish, and the bottom part becomes reddish because of hemorrhaging. Death can result.

Metals are still other chemicals that poison in numerous ways. A case history from Singapore illustrates one mode of attack. A laborer was admitted to a hospital with various symptoms—loss of weight, abscesses all over his body, nausea, vomiting, kidney and nervous system damage. Just before he died the cause was discovered. He had been at a bazaar and had agreed to let a medicine man inject quicksilver into his body to cure

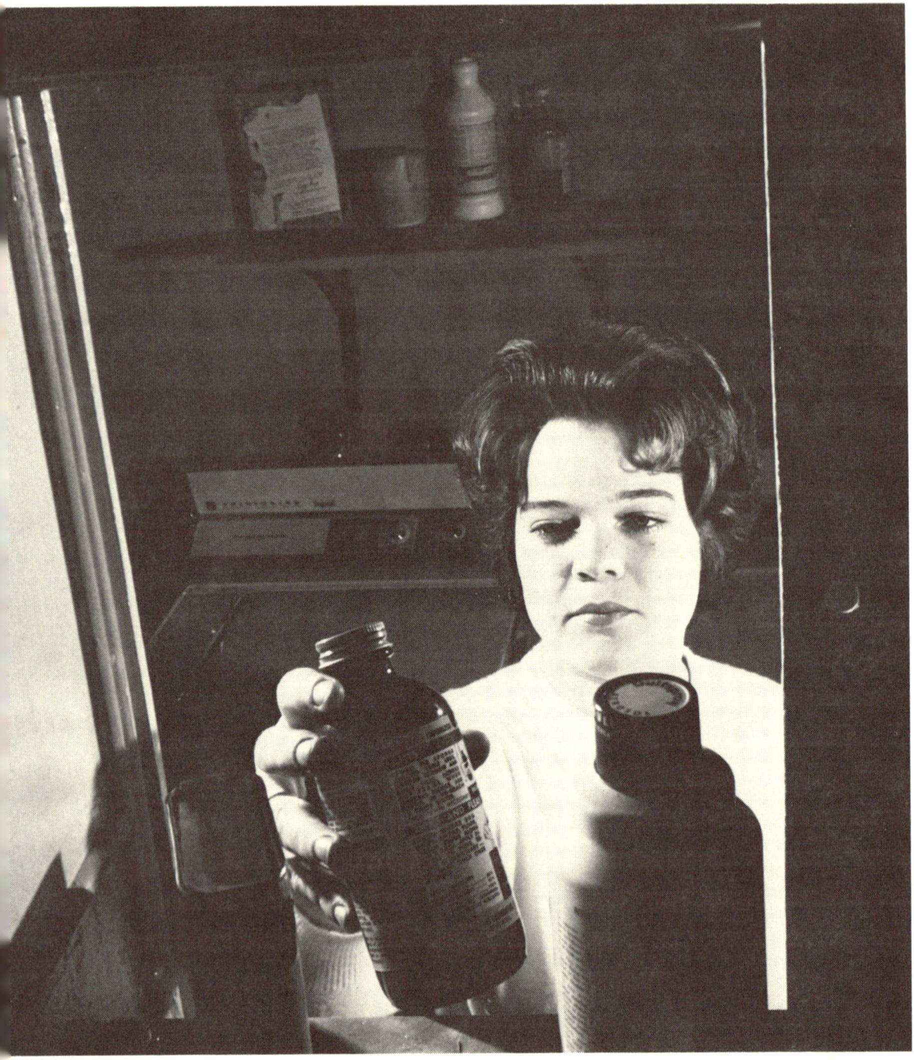

U. S. DEPARTMENT OF AGRICULTURE

Dangerous household chemicals such as carbolic acid, lye, ammonia, furniture polish, turpentine, insecticides, mothballs, and all drugs and ointments should be kept only in high closets out of reach of children and pets.

him of diabetes. What the laborer didn't know is that quicksilver is nothing less than the metallic element mercury, which is highly poisonous.

Antimony, on the other hand, injures the heart and leads to heart attacks. If iodine is swallowed, it burns the mouth and throat and leads to excessive thirst and vomiting. Lead exerts a multipronged attack. It interferes with acetylcholine and iron-containing enzymes in the blood so that hemoglobin cannot be made. It attacks the nuclei of cells and inhibits enzymes in the liver. Chronic lead poisoning, as in children who nibble lead paint, results in damage to the kidneys, blood vessels, and nervous system.

The initial symptoms of iron poisoning are vomiting, diarrhea, and lethargy, as seen in children who have swallowed large numbers of vitamin pills loaded with iron. Some of these youngsters have gone on to suffer low blood sugar, liver and kidney damage, and death. In severe arsenic poisoning, the heart, kidneys, and other organs are damaged. Then comes vomiting, diarrhea, abdominal pain, and death. Arsenic can take several hours to several days to kill. Arsenic poisoning, however, may be less severe, leading to simply loss of weight and skin rashes.

As for drugs and household products that can poison, aspirin damages the kidneys and leads to fever, hemorrhage, confusion, convulsions, coma, and death. If ammonia water is drunk, it burns the mouth and throat. Rat poisons lead to convulsions and stoppage of breathing. Mothballs produce nausea, depression, coma, convulsions, and death within a few hours to a few days.

Thousands and Thousands of Chemicals

On the whole, the nonbiological toxins present a far greater challenge to scientists than do the biological toxins. The reason is simply that they are so numerous —hundreds of thousands of industrial chemicals, 50,000 drugs, 36,000 pesticides, 7000 food additives— and everywhere in the environment. The challenge consists in answering a number of pressing questions. For instance, how many environmental chemicals interact with each other before they enter the body? Do such interactions increase their toxicity? Preliminary evidence suggests that they can. Can tissue culture and animal-study results really be guidance for the human condition, especially when extremely large doses of chemicals are used to achieve toxic effects? Scientists hope that they can, but they aren't sure. For instance, the defoliant 2,4,5-T was widely used to clear jungles and destroy crops in Vietnam during the Vietnam war. This chemical induces birth defects in mice and rats. But it has never been proven that the chemical induced any birth defects in Vietnamese children.

How long do various compounds stay in the body? In what forms? Perhaps the reason that Kepone produces long-range deleterious effects in people and that DDT does not is that the latter quickly breaks down in the body to the less toxic DDE. Do compounds interact in the body and produce even more poisonous effects than they would alone? Preliminary studies suggest that they do. Aspirin, for example, has been found to interact with alcohol, vitamin C, and several other drugs, leading to toxic complications. Commonly used alkalizing tablets interfere with antacids, vitamins and antibiotics, also leading to complex toxic interactions. Nose drops that interact with digitalis, aspirin, cold tablets, and blood-pressure-lowering drugs, likewise create toxicity. Pesticides and various drugs may also aggravate each other's toxicity in the body.

Individual susceptibility to toxic chemicals is still another area that scientists want to explore more. Extremely old and young persons appear to be particularly vulnerable, as do those who have not inherited all the liver enzymes necessary for breaking down and disposing of foreign chemicals in the body. Nutrition also appears to influence liver enzymes and how well they dispose of chemicals. Stress does too.

And then there is the urgent question of whether toxicity can be equated with causing cancer. Substantial evidence suggests that in some cases it can. For example, some of the victims of the atomic bombing in Japan subsequently came down with leukemia. In 1972 the Environmental Protection Agency banned the use of DDT, not so much because it posed a toxic hazard to people but principally because it triggered cancer in lab animals, thereby suggesting that it might cause cancer in humans. In 1975 the EPA decided that the pesticides heptachlor and chlordane should come off the market because they started cancer going in lab animals. In 1976 Hopewell, Virginia residents who had been found to have Kepone in their blood waited in anguish to see whether they might develop liver cancer, because the National Cancer Institute had just found that the pesticide causes liver cancer in laboratory animals.

Other evidence, though, suggests that toxic chemicals do not always cause the disease. The NCI studied some 80 pesticides and found that only one-sixth of them brought on cancer in test animals. In 1975 the medical community feared that astronaut Donald K. (Deke) Slayton was developing lung cancer from breathing poisonous nitrogen tetroxide fumes from rocket fuel. It turned out that he was not.

Still other evidence shows that some compounds that cause cancer are not particularly toxic, again suggesting that toxicity cannot always be equated with causing cancer. For instance, beta naphthylamine, which produces bladder cancer in industrial workers, isn't very toxic.

What's Being Done?

So while scientists are attempting to answer these numerous and incredibly complex questions about environmental chemicals, government agencies, the medical profession, and Congress are, on the whole, attempting to protect people against their toxic effects. And they are making some progress in that direction. For instance, the Food and Drug Administration has been imposing increasingly stringent requirements for the testing of new drugs to make sure that they are not toxic or cancer-causing. The requirements are so strict and time-consuming, in fact, that certain critics charge the FDA with keeping valuable new drugs off the market.

The EPA has analyzed the drinking water of 80 cities for carbon tetrachloride, chloroform, and other toxic compounds. Scientists at the National Bureau of Standards have developed a sensitive monitor for determining the occupational exposure of workers to mercury over a workday. The American Society for Experimental Pathology is studying suspect industrial chemicals, pesticides, food additives, and drugs to see whether they cause cancer. It is using a new technique developed by Dr. Joseph DiPaolo that may indicate cancer-causation in as little as two weeks. The chemical companies may gradually be showing somewhat more responsibility, if a 1975 development produces valid results. In that year the Chemical Industry Institute of Toxicology got off the ground, thanks to underwriting by major chemical companies. The institute was set up to assess the safety of chemicals being used for a number of purposes. Members of Congress are pushing for a toxic-substances act that would require testing of all chemicals before they are used.

Meanwhile there are serious gaps in efforts to protect

the public from poisonous substances. Federal laws dealing with toxic chemicals are piecemeal and haphazard. Many such substances are not subject to effective regulation even though their hazards may be known. And tragedies like that at Hopewell, Virginia, continue to happen because workers weren't informed of the toxicity of the chemical they were working with and weren't provided with adequate safety equipment. The workers blamed the chemist and the manager of the Life Science Products Company. The chemist and manager in turn blamed Allied Chemical Company, which had contracted Kepone production to Life Science. Allied managers in turn blamed the chemist and manager at Life Science.

So who was really to blame? No one is sure; it may be a long time before the culprits are uncovered. Meanwhile workers at other plants and residents in other American towns are probably encountering comparable risks, and the government and industries aren't finding it any easier to protect them, as the hundreds of thousands of chemicals in air, food, and water are joined by 200,000 new ones each year.

7 · Poisons in Murders and Suicides

During World War I, the Hungarian villages of Nagyrév and Tiszakürt fell into what some might call a state of moral decline. All but the very young and very old men were off fighting, so the village women, deprived of their husbands and lovers, turned to village war prisoners for company. These women grew so fond of their new freedoms, in fact, that they were sorry to see their husbands and lovers return from war.

One drab autumn day Mrs. Ilona G. of Nagyrév had a flash of inspiration. She called on Mrs. Nora F., a red-haired, green-eyed resident of Tiszakürt and a woman of notorious shrewdness and cunning. Mrs. F. already had a lucrative abortion trade under way. "Tell me, Nora," Mrs. G. asked, "can you help me get rid of Imre? I honestly cannot tolerate him any longer."

"But of course, Ilona," Mrs. F. replied with a smile. "For enough forints [Hungarian money] I can help you do anything."

Mrs. F. then deftly set about removing arsenic from

flypaper and mixed it into a spicy Hungarian goulash. "Here, feed that to Imre," she commanded. Mrs. G. did as told. Within two days Mr. G. was dead.

Quietly, discreetly, word of Mr. G.'s demise spread among other discontented women in Nagyrév and Tiszakürt: "Did you hear how Ilona got rid of Imre?" Soon other women also sought Mrs. F.'s assistance. Within several months a Tiszakürt husband drank a sweet Hungarian wine and died. Three weeks later a Nagyrév husband downed a vial of gout medicine and succumbed. Year after year husbands in Nagyrév and Tiszakürt quietly went to their graves. Mrs. F. became a very rich woman.

Finally in 1924, a good decade later, the tide turned against Mrs. F. and her clientele. A bright young doctor who had just finished his medical training in Budapest moved to Nagyrév to practice. Suspecting that one of his patients had been poisoned with arsenic, he requested an autopsy. Several villagers who had not participated in the poisonings but who knew about them sent anonymous letters to the local authorities. The authorities took action and demanded that the bodies of hundreds of husbands who had died during the previous 10 years be exhumed. Eighty-six of them were found to contain large amounts of arsenic, indicating that they had been poisoned. Mrs. F. was accused of the crimes. But on the eve of her arrest she boasted, "They'll never get me!" She drank a caustic alkali and died.

This true account of Mrs. F., one of the most notorious poisoners of modern times, shows that the real-life role of poisons in murders can be every bit as dramatic as those whipped up by mystery writers such as Agatha Christie (being a pharmacist, she often used poisons as murder weapons in her books); Joseph Otto Kesselring (author of the famous melodrama *Arsenic and Old Lace*); John Dickson Carr (author of *Poison in Jest*), and Charlotte Armstrong (author of *A Dram of Poison*).

Thinking Out the Murder

Indeed, if there is anything that unites cases of murder by poisoning throughout history with those of fiction, it is the nature of the murders and murderers. Unlike most murders, those by poisoning are invariably premeditated, declares Dr. James P. Weston, a medical examiner in New Mexico. Dr. Irving Sunshine, a forensic toxicologist in Cleveland, agrees: "A poisoning has to be by definition a premeditated thing." Examples of such can be found among the Borgias and Rasputin's murderer, as mentioned in Chapter 1. The famous "Affair of the Poisons" in seventeenth-century France was another. A three-year investigation revealed that nobles, prosperous bourgeois, and even commoners were regularly purchasing poisons for criminal purposes. The investigation led to 319 arrests and 36 poisoners' being sentenced to death.

Homicidal poisonings are usually motivated by some of humanity's basest feelings—hatred, greed, revenge, or simply the sheer love of murder. A prime example of hatred motivating homicidal poisonings can be found, of course, among the women of Nagyrév and Tiszakürt. A good example of greed comes from the eighteenth century. A sea captain married a young woman for her dowry. But it was not enough to satisfy him. Since her brother's estate would fall to them if the brother died, the captain decided to poison him. He mixed a solution of cherry laurel taken from the garden and got the brother to drink it. Within ten minutes the brother's stomach rattled, his teeth clenched, and he fell over dead. The captain was found guilty and executed.

The 1950s saw another major homicidal poisoning prompted by greed. A hard-boiled Britisher, Mrs. Margaret M., was caring for an old lady. Since her charge had willed her bungalow and few worldly possessions to Mrs. M., her companion decided to poison her. In fact, Mrs. M. was so anxious to inherit the old lady's possessions that she boasted even before she carried out her deed that she would soon acquire them. Mrs. M. was convicted of the murder and hung.

If there was ever a prime instance of homicidal poisoning being committed for the lust of it, it was in the nineteenth century. A nurse living in Leiden, Holland, killed 27 persons with poison and attempted to do in 75 more. She was finally apprehended.

A common characteristic of poisoners is that they

are bright, coolly logical, and far from insane, although one might well accuse them of having warped minds. Putting all the aspects of homicidal poisonings and poisoners together—premeditation, motivations of the lowest order, and a smart, logical mind—it's hardly surprising that they fill most members of society with chills and foreboding and have great appeal for mystery writers and mystery fans.

Poisonings Today and Yesterday

Still another intriguing aspect of homicidal poisonings both today and in earlier years is that the choice of poisons hasn't changed all that much, even though many more chemicals are available today. Why is this? "Poisoners often get their ideas from reading mysteries," Dr. Weston says. "That is why arsenic and strychnine still occur so frequently in homicidal poisoning." However, some newer poisons are used today too, such as thallium (a rat poison), succinylcholine (a drug that resembles curare), pesticides, and weed-killers. A medical examiner in London is currently investigating a murder by the weed-killer paraquat. Then there is chloral hydrate, which is used as lethal knockout drops.

If there is one thing that is strikingly different about homicidal poisonings today compared with yesterday, though, it is that they are far less common today than in the past centuries. The reasons, however, are not particularly obvious. One might assume that one reason is

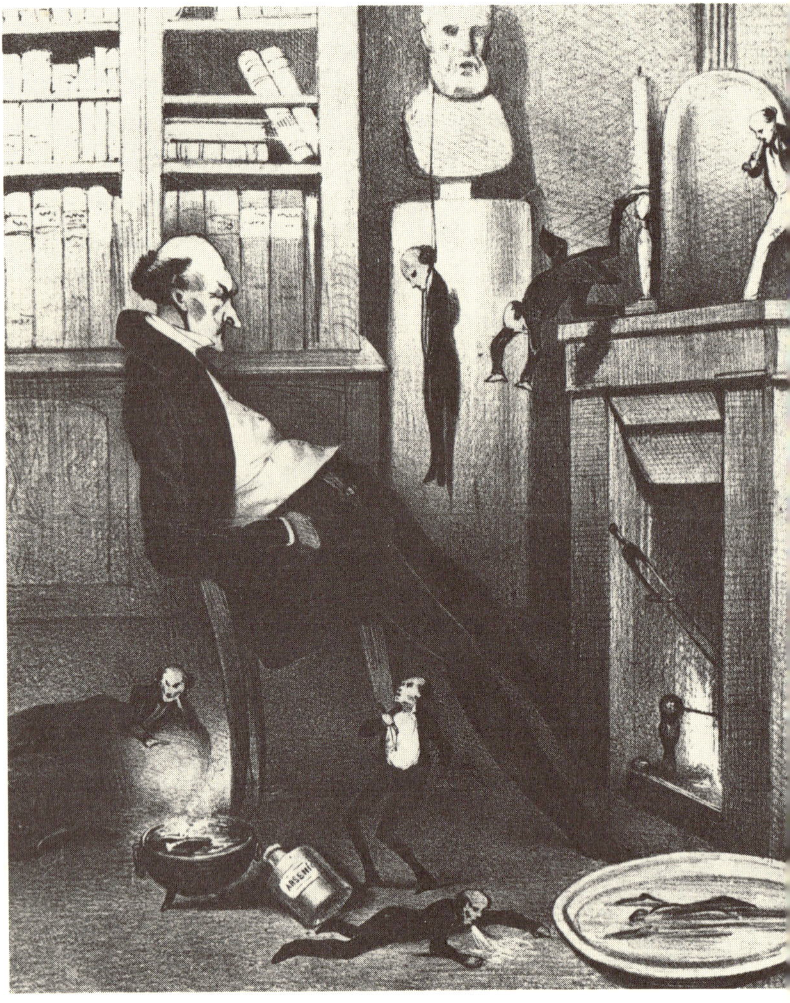

NATIONAL LIBRARY OF MEDICINE

In this almost surrealist lithograph the noted artist Honoré Daumier dealt with the tragic subject of suicide, through the imaginings of an unhappy middle-aged man. One of the suicidal methods envisioned is the use of arsenic, in the bottle on the floor; another is the inhalation of poisonous fumes. The picture was published in 1833 in the French magazine Le Charivari.

that there are stricter laws now against the purchase of poisons. But Dr. Abraham Stolman, a forensic toxicologist in Hartford, Connecticut, doesn't think so. "Today you can go into any garden store," he says, "and you can buy all the arsenic you want." Might the main reason be that medical examiners and forensic toxicologists are better at detecting poisons in the bodies of victims and hence frighten off potential poisoners? Dr. Weston thinks so. But Dr. Stolman disagrees: "I don't think the sophistication of techniques has anything to do with fewer homicidal poisonings. We just detect them more readily, that is all." Dr. Sunshine agrees with Dr. Stolman: "No, I don't think that the fact that techniques are far more advanced today than they ever were before has anything to do with poisons being used less today than before." The reasons remain obscure.

The Tragedy of Suicide

One thing that medical examiners and forensic toxicologists do agree on, though, is that suicides by poisoning are extremely frequent today. And again the reasons are not obvious. According to a report in a 1974 issue of the British medical journal *Lancet*, suicidal poisoning attempts are particularly common among teenagers and even becoming more frequent. When teenagers attempt to poison themselves, the article said, it is usually because they are from unhappy homes, lack self-esteem, and have just had a falling-out with people who are important in their lives. Such disagreements can be over either major or trivial matters. For instance, a 17-year-old girl poisoned herself after she had a row with her family. Her father had had a stroke and couldn't work. The mother had to work in his place, yet suggested it was the girl's role to assume the family's financial burdens. The girl felt trapped and did away with herself. In contrast, a 16-year-old girl poisoned herself for a far less important reason. She had fought with her boy friend over the way his hair had been cut.

The types of poisons used in suicide today "vary with the going vogue," Dr. Sunshine says. "It's a question of what's available." Overdoses of drugs such as aspirin, barbiturates, tranquilizers, and antidepressants are chosen often. And an article in a 1975 issue of the *American Medical Association News* reported that an overdose of Darvon—a prescription pain reliever second only to aspirin in popularity—is becoming extremely common as a suicidal agent. Dr. Stolman agrees: "One of the big problems today is that we are seeing an increase of death rates from Darvon." The reason, apparently, is that physicians prescribe Darvon freely, not realizing that 15 to 20 capsules are enough to cause death and even fewer capsules are needed if they are combined with alcohol.

Although carbon monoxide is not used as a suicidal agent as much today as a few years ago, due to a change in the composition of domestic gas, it is still used. Pesticides and herbicides are also common suicide agents today. For instance, a 51-year-old man took three ounces of paraquat in a suicide attempt and was dead three days later. A 58-year-old woman took it to commit suicide. She was admitted to the hospital eight days later. And a week after that she died. Then a 64-year-old widow, depressed and sick, drank the herbicide sodium chlorate. She lived for a week with no other symptoms than extreme depression. Then she became

Carbon monoxide affects red blood cells, seen here, by chemically binding to the hemoglobin in them, which prevents the hemoglobin from carrying oxygen to the tissues. Carbon monoxide comes from incomplete burning, appearing, for instance, in smoke from cigarettes and exhaust from cars. In sufficient quantities it can kill; even driving a car in traffic can cause the driver to lose alertness and misjudge distances—especially if he is smoking also. MARCH OF DIMES

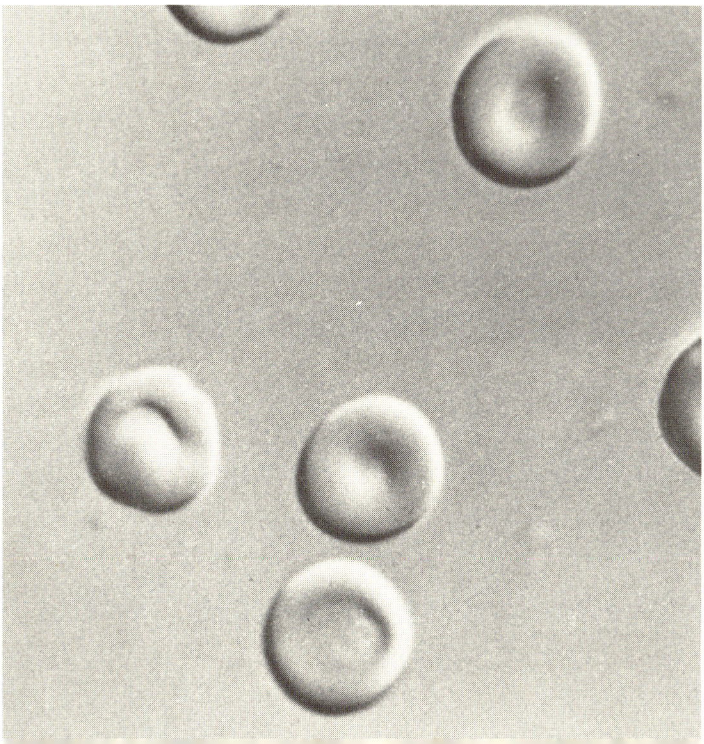

unconscious and was taken to the hospital. The physicians thought that she had taken an overdose of barbiturates and treated her accordingly. So she died. Upon autopsy they discovered the real reason for her death. Her lips had a cyanide tinge, her back was livid, and her blood was a brownish color. Sodium chlorate was present in her urine.

Help From the Laboratory

Precisely what progress has science made in detecting poisons in the bodies of victims and in helping the law determine whether they are homicidal or suicidal? Methods started to develop some 200 years ago. Ways of detecting arsenic in victims became available in the eighteenth century. But they weren't always reliable. Then a British chemist, James Marsh, came up with a better method in 1832. The intestines of a poisoned man, together with the contents of a coffee pot, were delivered to Marsh for analysis. Both yielded a yellow precipitate, which indicated arsenic. But the accused was acquitted. The jurors simply did not have faith in scientific advancement. They wanted to see the "real arsenic," which meant to them a white powder.

His pride stung, Marsh set out to find another, more convincing test for arsenic. He made a U-shaped glass tube, with one end open and the other terminating in the nozzle in which he suspended a piece of zinc. Then he introduced into the tube a sample of the material to be tested with either hydrochloric or sulfuric acid. When the mixture reached the zinc, hydrogen was liberated. The hydrogen then reacted with any arsenic present to form arsine gas, which escaped through the nozzle. When the arsine was ignited, black metallic arsenic deposited itself in a bowl held above the nozzle.

This test was better accepted by jurors, but still trouble arose. Arsenic was found in the bones of persons who had died from natural causes. But finally this problem was overcome. If considerable amounts of arsenic were in the ground around a coffin, then one would have to expect some of it to make its way into a corpse, in which case the presence of arsenic would not necessarily indicate homicidal or suicidal poisoning.

Tests for detecting lethal levels of other inorganic materials in the body were also developed in the nineteenth century, for antimony, lead, mercury, sulfur. Then another challenge arose for forensic medicine: the expanding use of plant toxins in homicides and suicides. There was no way to detect their presence in the tissues of victims. The prosecutor at one trial for a morphine murder said bitterly: "So, murderers, use plant poisons to kill your fathers, your mothers, your entire families. Fear not; your crimes will go unpunished." Finally in 1863 a technique was successfully devised to detect digitalis poisoning, and a murderer was convicted on the basis of it. And in 1882 aconite was detected in the body of a victim, and the murderer was convicted.

By 1914 forensic toxicologists were regularly able to

detect the presence of plant toxins in victims by the use of a technique called X-ray diffraction, in which X rays bounce off the atoms of a crystal to form distinctive patterns. Crystals of the toxins could be identified from two diffraction patterns on a photographic plate. Toward the late 1940s two far more valuable techniques became available for testing all sorts of poisons. They were spectrometry and chromatography. These methods are capable of separating almost any poison in body tissues or fluids from other chemicals that might be present and determining the molecular configuration of the poison. In that way the poison can be identified.

Today forensic scientists use essentially the same techniques, but with the equipment hooked up to a computer, which checks chromatograph and spectrometer findings against a vast collection of poisons. The computer can say not only whether a person's body contains this or that poison and in what concentration. It can even tell whether any breakdown products of the poisons are present in the body. And it can detect poisons in incredibly small amounts. "At one time," Dr. Stolman says, "we were lucky if we could detect a milligram of a poison. Now we can detect a thousandth of a milligram or a millionth of a milligram."

Still another technique forensic scientists have acquired in the past 10 years is the immunoassay, in which antibodies to specific poisons can be used to identify the smallest traces of a poison in blood. In an Oradell, New Jersey, hospital six patients died mysteriously from suspected poisoning in 1966. The cases were closed later with no one accused of the murders. They were reopened in 1976 and an immunoassay on the corpses exhumed from 10 years before showed that curare, the suspected poison, was present.

Thus the latest scientific detection methods help immensely in leading to the prosecution of homicidal poisoners and in clearing of suspicion families and friends of suicides. Nonetheless, the scientists still find room for progress. The problem, Dr. Weston explains, is that homicidal and suicidal poisonings are not always suspected. "The toxicologist," he says, "is not so sophisticated, nor is the community so well endowed, that we can take a blood sample on all people who die and run it through one of these machines. We don't have enough of the machines, we don't have enough toxicologists. I think the key part of the investigation boils down to whether there is a possibility that the person was killed by a poison." For instance, was a poison found in food, drink, or other material left near the victim or in the victim's household? If so, then investigators would have reason to suspect a homicidal or suicidal poison and would call in forensic scientists.

Even if such researchers were able to detect all homicidal and suicidal poisonings, it would hardly stop such poisonings from occurring. Here it is a question not of science but of society as a whole. If people really want to murder, they'll find some way to do it. If people really want to kill themselves, they'll go to astonishing lengths to do so. For instance, the 51-year-old man who finally killed himself with paraquat had previously attempted to kill himself with gas, codeine tablets, and by slashing his wrists. The 64-year-old widow who finally managed to kill herself with sodium chlorate had tried to kill herself before with two other chemicals.

"During the next 20 years poisons will not be used extensively for homicides," Dr. Sunshine predicts. "But they will be used continually by people intent on suicides, because they are available and because people have been educated that this is an easy way to do things."

8 · Poisons in Warfare

April 22, 1915, was a day unprecedented in history. Allied troops were hiding in trenches in Ypres, France. They heard a hissing noise from the German trenches. Within 15 minutes, 168 tons of chlorine were released along the four-mile front. A ghoulish green mist invaded the Allied trenches. The deadly gas filled the soldiers with horror and confusion. Those who could fled past rear positions, only to run the risk of being shot by comrades who were unaware of the advancing terror. More chlorine was discharged on the Allies two days later, along with shells of tear gas. Five thousand soldiers were killed, 10,000 suffered gas effects and wounds.

These two days in World War I mark the first extensive, successful use of poisons in warfare. True, poisons had been tried before, but on a more modest scale. In 600 B.C., for example, the Athenian legislator Solon had roots of hellebore thrown into a small river, which the enemy used for drinking water. It led to a violent attack of diarrhea and the enemy's

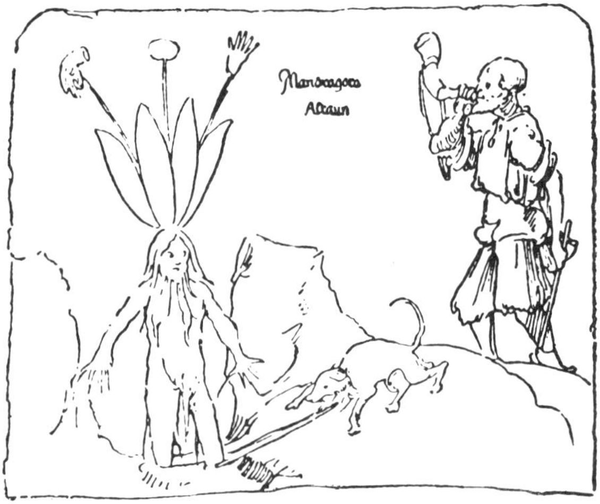

Mandragora, the mandrake plant, has been in use since ancient times as a toxin that causes deep sleep; it was one of the first anesthetics, being used for operations by an army surgeon serving Nero. This medieval picture shows popular superstitions of the time: that a mandrake plant resembled a human being, and that it shrieked on being pulled from the ground, causing anyone hearing it to go mad. Thus the man stood at a distance, using a dog to gather the plant, and blew a horn to drown out any sound that reached him.

defeat. Then in 200 B.C. a Carthaginian general put roots of mandragora into the wine of an enemy. The roots made the enemy fall into a drugged sleep, so that he and his soldiers could kill them. During the eleventh century Emperor Frederick Barbarossa conquered an Italian town by poisoning its water supply with carcasses.

1915: Tragic Year

The reason that the age of poisons in warfare didn't come about until World War I was principally that scientists hadn't known nearly as much about the chemistry of poisons before then. Nor had they been in a position to synthesize potent poisons, and in large quantities. Consequently, 1915 was just a start in the age of poisons in warfare. More efforts at poisoning were to come in the subsequent months of World War I.

Soon the Allies were retaliating aganst the Germans with chlorine and designing protective masks for themselves. Then the Germans introduced an even more toxic gas, phosgene. Once again the Allies designed protection against it and used phosgene too. The Germans then introduced two even more deadly chemicals —diphenylchloroarsine, a cough-inducing agent, and mustard gas, which is really not a gas, but an oily liquid that inflicts death by skin contact. The Allies did the same.

By World War II, the specter of poisons in warfare was even larger. Pesticide research, for example, had led to the invention of nerve gases, which are far more dangerous than even mustard gas. They are truly weapons of mass destruction. Both the Germans and Allies had isolated botulism toxin in pure form. But none of the European powers nor the United States used these or any other poison during the war. There were several reasons. Opposing forces feared the threat of retaliation. The military was skeptical about their utility. And, most critically, there was a widespread abhorrence toward using gases and germs in warfare. All the major European powers had signed the Geneva Protocol by 1939. And while the United States had not signed it, President Roosevelt still declared that gas warfare was "outlawed by the general opinion of civilized mankind" and that "we shall under no circumstances resort to the use of such weapons unless they are first used by our enemies."

The 1950s did not bring about any major uses of poison in war. But this decade saw major powers, including the United States, stockpiling poisons in the event that they might later decide to use them. The United States, for example, set up Edgewood Arsenal and Fort Detrick in Maryland, Pine Bluff Arsenal in Arkansas, and Rocky Mountain Arsenal in Colorado to develop and stockpile poisons as weapons. Scientists at these arsenals developed large batches of botulism toxin, cobra toxin, saxitoxin, and a plague more deadly than the Black Death, which killed one-fourth of the human race during the Middle Ages.

Assassination Attempts, Herbicides, Phosgene

During the early 1960s, however, the United States attempted to use poisons secretly. The United States Army made saxitoxin and cobra toxin caches available

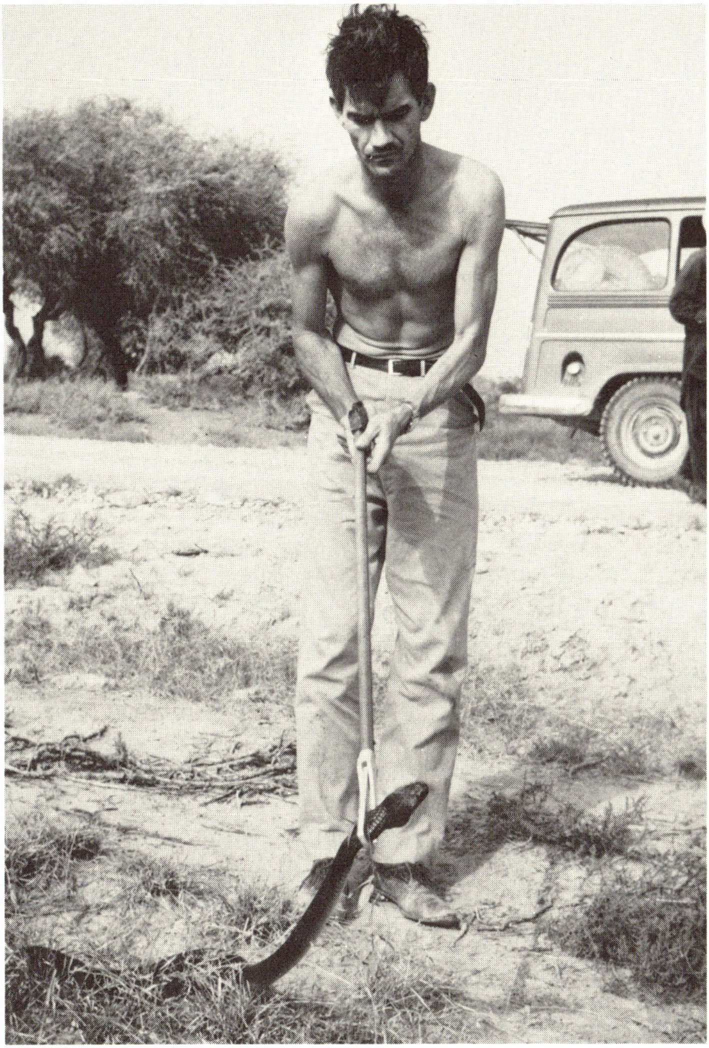

DR. SHERMAN A. MINTON

Cobras, like this one being caught near Karachi, Pakistan, occur through much of Asia and Africa. Cobra toxin is one of the poisons with which the U. S. Army has experimented for possible use in chemical warfare.

to the Central Intelligence Agency. The CIA also attempted to poison several foreign leaders that it considered to be enemies of the United States, notably Cuban Premier Fidel Castro and Congolese Premier Patrice Lumumba. On November 22, 1963, the day President John Kennedy was killed in Dallas, a high-ranking CIA officer met with a secret Cuban agent. He gave the Cuban a poison pen rigged with a hypodermic needle to use on Castro. The pen, however, was not used. Then the CIA concocted some other plots to poison Castro, using poisonous cigars, exploding seashells, and a contaminated diving suit. But for one reason or another it never did manage to poison either Castro or Lumumba.

Several attempts at using poisons in the course of warfare did succeed during the 1960s and early 1970s. Between 1961 and 1971, the United States military dropped more than 100 million pounds of herbicides on the vegetation of Vietnam. The purpose was to wipe out the Vietcong's cover and destroy crops, with the hope of causing widespread starvation. The herbicides used were 2,4-5, 2,4,5-T, 2,4-D plus picloram (like DDT), and arsenic. During 1966 and 1967, the Egyptians used both mustard gas and phosgene on citizens of Yemen. Several hundred were killed.

Still other poisoning incidents and attempts have occurred during the twentieth century. But they haven't received as much publicity as those above. In fact, there have probably been more incidents and attempts than most of us realize, because they haven't worked out or because they have been kept secret by the governments involved.

Poisons in Warfare: the Debate

There are several strong reasons for using poisons in warfare, a number of generals and scientists have argued. One is that poisons tend to incapacitate victims but not kill them. For instance, the ratio of deaths to casualties due to poisonous warfare during World War I may have been as low as 7 per cent, whereas it was 25 per cent for conventional weapons. Still another argument for poisonous weapons is that if they do kill, they are quicker and less painful than conventional weapons. In 1942, for instance, the American Brigadier General Alden H. Waitt admitted that nerve gases might trigger a larger proportion of deaths and more suffering than gases used in World War I. But he argued that they still wouldn't approach conventional weapons in their devastating effects. Still another proponent of poisonous weapons asked: "Do you think that the bayonet is more humane than gas? Men are trained to stick it in the belly and twist it around, thus causing painful injury and almost certain death after prolonged agony. Are high explosives and shrapnel humane? Think of the torn and mangled bodies."

Those who argue against the use of poisons in warfare, however, point out that gases used in World War I did more than temporarily incapacitate soldiers. Men exposed to even lower doses of chlorine, they say, experienced a burning of the throat and suffocation, death often following after two days. Or, as the British writer Conan Doyle observed in 1915: the chlorine attack on the Allied troops at Ypres left "dead garrisons, whose blackened faces, contorted figures and lips fringed with blood and foam from their bursting lungs, showed the agonies in which they had died." Then in 1917, the opponents of poisonous weapons continue, British soldiers attacked by mustard gas vomited, and those without eye protection became blind. Some of the soldiers' lungs practically disintegrated. Those who were fortunate enough to be removed from the front sometimes took months to recover, meanwhile experiencing headache, nausea, and intense depression. As for the nerve gases, they inactivate cholinesterase and lead to blurred vision, intense salivation, convulsions, and death through suffocation.

Aside from the use of poisons in combat, the opponents continue, consider their use under other conditions. During the 1950s and 1960s, for instance, the U. S. Army gave the hallucinogen LSD to thousands of soldiers, some of whom volunteered for the test. The Army was contemplating using LSD as an offensive weapon and wanted to learn more about its effects on soldiers. However, the Army failed to tell the nonvolunteer subjects what they had been given or how it might affect them; in fact, they didn't know they were receiving any drug whatever. The testing resulted in one case of suicide and two soldiers' developing convulsive seizures. Until 1974 the Army was also testing the chemical BZ on soldiers. It can trigger unpredictable and violent behavior. Again at least some of the subjects were not told what they were getting or what they might expect from it.

There is also the danger, opponents of poisonous warfare assert, that poisons intended for soldiers will hurt civilians. In 1943 mustard gas was on an American ship that accidentally blew up off the coast of Italy. The result was 617 casualties. Despite safety measures, several researchers at Fort Detrick, Maryland, died from poisons they were concocting. During the late 1960s accidental release of a nerve gas at a U. S. military base in Japan injured 24 persons. On March 13, 1968, an Air Force jet roared over the Utah desert and sprayed out 320 gallons of nerve gas. A valve on the dispenser had failed to snap shut. The deadly gas continued to pour from the airplane and was carried 45 miles away from the target area. Within three days, 6400 sheep in Skull and Rush Valleys died as a result. Salt Lake City was 380 miles from the target area. Although extensive investigation has not proven that the defoliant 2,4,5-T caused birth defects among the Vietnamese people, it may still have exerted subtle forms of brain and nervous damage on their offspring. The chemical has been found to cause birth defects in laboratory animals.

Treaties Kept and Treaties Broken

What will the future bring as far as the use of poisons in warfare is concerned? Treaties banning the use of poisons have been signed by countries in the past and have deterred the use of poisonous weapons to some degree. For instance, Germany, Britain, and France signed the Geneva Protocol of 1925 banning the use of poisons. They abided by the protocol throughout World War II. But treaties haven't countered the use of poisons in other instances. Although the major powers had agreed before World War I not to use poisons, they ended up using them anyway. Then, during the 1960s, the United States said it was adhering to the Geneva Protocol while it dropped herbicides on Vietnam, saying that herbicides didn't fall under the protocol. But other countries insisted it did. Britain in 1970 took a position similar to that of the United States, stating that certain irritant gases such as tear gas are not covered by the protocol. In that way she could use these gases in northern Ireland.

Even if governments wish to adhere to treaties against the use of poisonous weapons, certain government factions may resist. In late 1969 and early 1970, President Richard Nixon proclaimed that the United States would never be the first to use lethal or incapacitating chemical or biological poisons. Under this new policy, the United States was to destroy stocks of microbes and microbial toxins and to stop their development and stockpiling. Research on microbial toxins was to be restricted to research for defensive purposes only, such as immunization. But in late 1975 the Congress learned that the Central Intelligence Agency had retained a secret cache of shellfish toxin and other deadly poisons that should have been destroyed five years earlier. The poisons were enough to kill thousands of persons.

What happened, apparently, was that the White House order, relayed orally down the ranks by the CIA director, bounced at the middle level. A chemist familiar with the difficulties of isolating toxins decided on his own to lock the supply away in case it might be wanted in the future. When he was asked during Congressional hearings in 1975 to explain his actions, he replied that he had not believed that the 1969 and 1970 presidential directives applied to the CIA and, second, that they applied to microbes, not to microbial toxins.

"Playing With Poisons"

The more important question, however, is why the CIA got into the poisons business in the first place. The *Washington Star* replied to this question in a 1975 editorial: "It may be that the CIA got into poisons because, in secret agencies, grown men like to play with poisons —especially if the curse can be taken off the word by calling them 'toxic substances.'" Certainly there is something to what the editorial says. The Congress learned, during its 1975 hearings into CIA activities, that the CIA had used the New York subways during the mid-1960s to stage simulated poison and germ attacks. CIA agents had also developed poisonous dart guns concealed in canes and umbrellas, exploding aerosol cans and gas-filled light bulbs. The guns included a .45 caliber-sized electric gun capable of silently firing poison pellets that would dissolve in a victim before an autopsy could be performed.

Governments like to state that they will not use poisonous weapons until the enemy does first. But they continue stockpiling such weapons. When Nixon banned the development of microbial toxins in 1969 and 1970, for instance, he did not do the same for the development of poisonous chemicals. The United States has continued to stockpile a variety of nerve-gas weapons that are thousands of times more potent than those of World War I. These gases kill when they are inhaled or when they are deposited as liquid droplets on the skin. Although BZ is not regarded as an ideal weapon, the U. S. Army still has it on hand. The Army has also found a new chemical known as EA-3834. It is classified and in the final stages of development. The United States is not the only nation building up its poisonous weapons, of course. The Soviet Union is doing the same.

As if the military isn't already dazzled enough with the poisons now at its disposal, it is doing work on making even more potent ones. For instance, the U. S. Army is now making binary weapons. They consist of comparatively innocuous chemicals separated from each other within a munition. At delivery, the chemicals mix, forming a poison such as nerve gas. The Army hopes eventually to have a billion-dollar binary weapons program. It argues that these weapons are safer to store and transport than ordinary chemical weapons are. Critics of binaries, however, charge that they are less efficient in battle than other chemicals and that their development is hindering poisons limitations agreements between the United States and the Soviet Union.

So a realistic conclusion about the future use of poisons as weapons in the world can only be as follows: treaties and limitations on the use of poisons in warfare should continue to be sought. They have helped deter deaths and misery by poisons in the past and will probably continue to do so in the future. But societies should not become complacent if agreements are reached. Rather, they should remain ever vigilant. Because as long as people have access to poisons, they will always be tempted to use them for destruction. That's human nature, as we know it up till now.

9 · Poisons and You

If anything has emerged from the previous chapters, it is that most of us don't have a whole lot of control over intentional efforts to poison us, whether they be homicidal poisoning or chemical warfare. However, we do have great control over accidental poisonings. So here are some suggestions on how to avoid them, and what to do if you or anyone near you is accidentally poisoned.

Avoiding Botulism

One of the best ways to avoid botulism, according to the U. S. Department of Agriculture, is to prepare home-processed foods properly. Before one cans low-acid foods, they should be pressure-cooked (how long depends on the kind of food and the size of the cooker). The reason is that a pressure cooker provides a heat of 240° F., which is higher than boiling temperature, and enough to kill botulinal spores. Without living spores, toxin cannot be produced. Before canning high-acid foods, such as tomatoes, one need only boil them; the reason being that botulinal spores will not normally grow in high-acid foods, but boiling is necessary to kill other organisms that might change the food into low-acid food and hence allow the spores to grow in it.

Before eating home-processed foods several months or more after preparation, boil them in a covered pot for at least ten minutes, even the acid ones (meat at least 20 minutes). In that way, if any botulinal spores did leave toxin behind, the toxin will be destroyed. In other words, precautions taken both before canning home-processed foods and before eating them provide double protection against botulism.

Since there are so few botulism outbreaks due to commercially prepared foods, it is not really necessary to boil commercially canned foods for a period of 10 minutes before eating, though boiling even these foods would give the highest possible protection. Frozen commercial foods should be kept frozen until cooking to prevent the growth of botulinal spores that could lead to production of the toxin.

For more information on safe methods of cooking, canning, and freezing foods, write for USDA bulletins on the subject, available from the Superintendent of Documents, U. S. Government Printing Office, Washington, D.C. 20402.

Foods in Countries With High Contamination

Some countries do not control their sanitary conditions as strictly as we may be used to. For instance, the biggest source of food poisoning in Mexico is fresh fruits and vegetables. If you go there, or anywhere with doubtful sanitation, don't eat them unless you peel those that are peelable; thoroughly cook all others. The way to keep from being poisoned by microbial toxins in drinking water in Mexico and many other countries is to drink carbonated water, tea, beer, or soft drinks instead of tap water. However, tap water can be made safe with water-purification tablets. Or you might want to do what Dr. Gangarosa does. He carries a little bottle of chlorine household bleach, such as Clorox, and uses an eyedropper to put one drop of it in a tall glass of water with no ice (which also can contain bacteria and toxins). After 15 minutes or so, the water should be safe to drink.

Children are more likely than adults to eat poisonous plants. So store bulbs and seeds safely away from children and pets; and label them. Teach children early to keep unknown plants and plant parts out of their mouths. Make them aware of the potential dangers of poisonous plants. Do not allow them to suck nectar from flowers or to make "tea" from leaves. As for yourself, don't eat wild plants or their fruits unless you can positively identify them as harmless. Avoid smoke from burning plants.

Mushrooms and Venoms

Children, on the other hand, are less likely than grownups to eat mushrooms, perhaps because they are

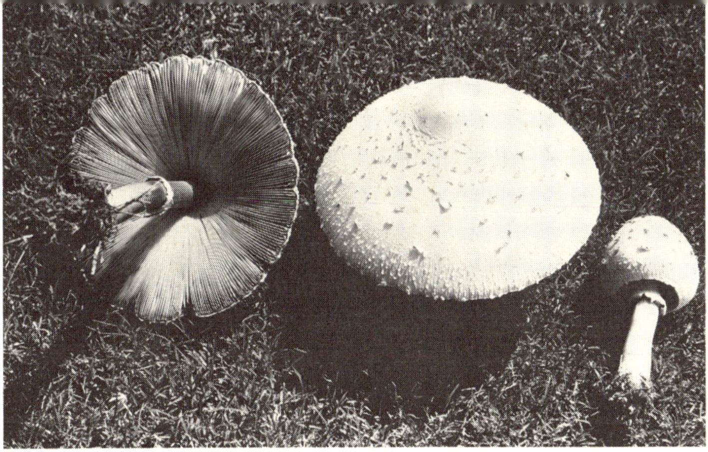

DR. L. F. GRAND

No wild mushroom should ever be eaten unless it is certified absolutely to be harmless. This is Morgan's mushroom (Lepiota morgani), *a species that can kill.*

less appealing to look at. Since harmless mushrooms often resemble highly toxic ones, get an expert's opinion before you attempt to eat *any* kind of wild mushroom. Don't believe old myths about mushroom identification, such as that edible mushrooms grow in a fairy ring, a piece of brass or silver will turn black if cooked with a poisonous fungus, or only edible species will peel. These ideas are false. Eating as little as one poisonous mushroom can make you seriously ill or even kill you.

If you're allergic to insect venoms, avoid using scented deodorants, hair sprays, and perfumes during the warm seasons, since the scent is attractive to some insects. Carry an insecticide spray in your pocket if working or playing out of doors. If you live in or visit an area where there are scorpions, wear heavy work gloves if cleaning up debris. If you feel something crawling over your body, don't swat it; brush it off. Swatting will guarantee poisoning, but a quick brush will remove the scorpion before it can sting.

Wear adequate clothing if you are hiking or camping in snake country—good, stout shoes and at least jeans to cover your legs. Be sure that you never put on shoes and clothing without shaking them out first. Don't leave your sleeping bag unrolled during the day. A snake might be hunting for a cool spot in which to pass the heat of midday. Establish camp early enough so you'll be settled before dark. This will give time to prepare a cleared space for beds and water. Stay on the trail. Watch where you put your hands and feet when climbing over logs, walls, etc. Never pick up an apparently

Rambling in the woods and fields is wonderful, but watch where you put your hands and where you sit. One of the many effects of carelessness can be poisoning from a spider bite, like this one from the brown spider Loxoceles laeta.

CENTER FOR DISEASE CONTROL, ATLANTA

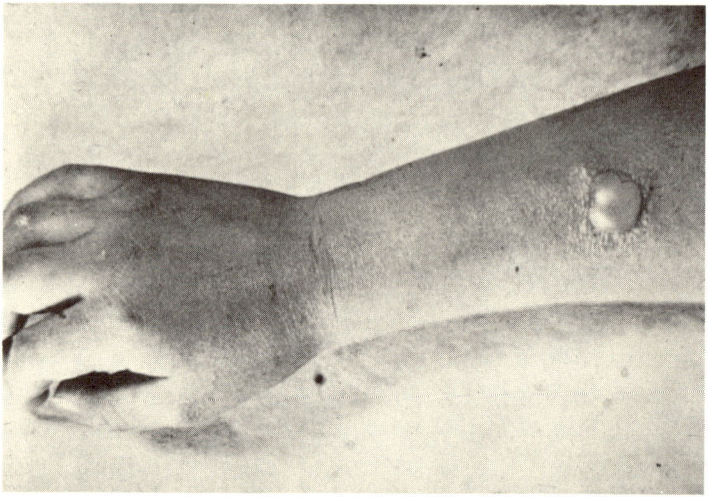

dead poisonous snake; there may be more life in it than you realize. Experiments have shown that a snake head severed from its body will remain alive and able to inflict a deadly bite for 15 to 30 minutes after being cut off.

If you are poisoned by microbes in food or water abroad, it probably won't be serious and will probably last four or five days at most. The crucial thing is to replace lost liquids—fruit juices with honey are ideal. Be wary of using foreign-made drugs abroad. They may do more harm than good.

In the case of plant poisoning, call your doctor or a local poison-control center immediately. Try to identify the species of plant that was eaten.

If someone is stung by an insect, remove the sting if possible. Apply ice, for cold slows chemical activity and retards absorption of venom. A few hours of ice treatment should be enough. Get the victim to a physician immediately if he has shortness of breath, generalized swelling, wheezing, abdominal pain, fainting, or shock.

First aid for scorpion bite, in all events, is to get the victim to a doctor or hospital. On the way, the victim's bitten hand or foot can be placed in ice water.

Snakebite

The most important first-aid measure against a poisonous snake bite is valuable only within the first 30 minutes after a bite. With a sterilized knife or razor blade, make an incision one-eighth or one-fourth inch in length over the fang marks. The incision should be made as deep as fang penetration. Suck out the poison through the incision. Do not use your mouth if another means of suction is available. Putting a tourniquet above the bite may also help. Keep the patient warm and get him to a hospital as quickly as possible for anti-venin therapy. Recent studies have shown that the anti-venin is most effective when given within four hours after a bite, and the earlier the better. It is of less value if delayed for eight hours and of questionable value after 24 hours.

If a person is bitten by a Gila monster, pry the animal loose from him quickly so as little venom as possible will be absorbed. Severe bleeding has been reported. A pressure dressing may hastily be applied to control hemorrhage. Get the victim to a doctor or hospital.

Victims of acid burns should have their burns covered with a clean cloth moistened with a warm solution of baking soda. Alkali burns, in contrast, should be neutralized with fruit juices. If a person has taken in a poisonous household product, try to identify the product and call your doctor or local poison-control center for advice on antidotes.

Before anything else, remember: prevention is always easier than cure.

Glossary

acetylcholine: A chemical released by nerves. It is crucial in nerve conduction.

alga: A primitive plant. Some can be seen with the naked eye, others only with a microscope. Many are harmless or even valuable to people, but some others make toxins that are poisonous to people.

alkaloid: A kind of chemical made by plants. A number are highly poisonous to humans.

amino acid: The chemical constituent of a protein.

antidote: An agent that neutralizes a poison or counters its effects.

antiserum: Blood containing antibodies against a poison.

antitoxin: An antibody formed in response to a toxin.

antivenin: An antiserum against an animal or insect venom.

atom: The smallest particle of an element that can exist alone or in combination.

bacterium: A microscopic, one-celled organism present in soil, water, plants, animals, and people. It may be harmless or even valuable to people or make toxins that are poisonous to them.

biotoxin: A biological poison; that is, a poison made by a living organism.

cholinesterase: An enzyme in the body that is vital for proper nerve conduction.

compound: A chemical substance formed by the union of two or more elements.

cyclic AMP: A crucial chemical messenger that operates inside cells.

dalton: A unit of measurement that scientists use to describe the weight of protein molecules and other molecules.

DNA: A nucleic acid that forms the genetic material of life; a gene is a section of a DNA molecule.

electron: One of the negative particles that make up an atom.

element: An aggregation of atoms of one kind only.

enzyme: A special class of proteins in cells that speed up chemical reactions without becoming a part of them.

forensic medicine: A special division of medical practice that assists murder trials and other legal proceedings.

fungus: A microbe that is sometimes considered a simple plant but is now usually classified by itself because it cannot make its own food. It can be harmless or even valuable to us, or it can make toxins that poison us.

glycoside: A class of plant chemical. A number are highly poisonous to humans. Some toads also make poisonous glycosides.

microbe: A microscopic organism.

molecule: The smallest possible quantity of a substance, usually made of two or more atoms, that retains the chemical properties of the substance.

nucleic acid: A complex acid found in cells.

oxalate: A class of chemical found in plants. Some are poisonous to people.

poison: A chemical that can harm the body if swallowed, inhaled, or absorbed through the skin. The term is usually reserved for a chemical that can kill when taken in very small amounts. The less it takes of a chemical to kill, the more poisonous it is considered.

platelet: A little platelike fragment in the blood that helps to clot it.

prostaglandin: A chemical that acts as a local hormonal messenger between cells.

protein: One of the most important classes of chemicals in plant, animal, and human cells. A number of animal proteins and a few plant proteins are poisonous.

RNA: A nucleic acid that translates a gene's information into protein manufacture.

saponin: A class of plant chemical. Some are poisonous to us. The sea star and sea cucumber also make toxic saponins.

toxic: Of, pertaining to, or caused by a poison or toxin.

toxicology: A science that deals with poisons and their effects on living organisms.

toxin: A term reserved for a poison from a living organism.

toxoid: A toxin that has been treated so that it is no longer toxic but still stimulates antibodies against itself and hence is valuable in vaccination.

venom: Poisonous material secreted by snakes, insects, and other animals.

Suggested Reading

Younger Books

Bessie M. Hecht, *Snakes* (Random House, 1956). All about snakes and their ways. The author also recalls her own experiences with snakes, such as milking venom from water moccasins.

Mary V. Hood, *Outdoor Hazards, Real and Fancied* (Macmillan, 1955). Ample information about poisonous animals in the United States, how to avoid being bitten by snakes, how to treat snakebites.

Robert M. McClung, *Buzztail; the Story of a Rattlesnake* (Morrow, 1958). One year in the life of Buzztail, a timber rattlesnakes, including its biting a careless farmboy.

John Perry, *Our Polluted World: Can Man Survive?* (Franklin Watts, 1972). Discusses pollution and what can be done about it. Includes pesticides, carbon monoxide poisoning, radioactive poisoning.

Dorothy Sterling, *The Story of Mosses, Ferns and Mushrooms* (Doubleday, 1955). Deals with what mushrooms are, how they grow, how they differ and warnings about poisonous mushrooms and false myths about them.

Louis Sutherland, *Magic Bullets* (Little, Brown, 1956). About the microbes that cause human disease and historical and modern attempts to control or destroy them.

Older and Adult Books

Joan Arehart-Treichel, *Immunity—How Our Bodies Resist Disease* (Holiday House, 1976). Takes up toxic microbes and how researchers and the human body fight them.

Dr. Melvin A. Benarde, *The Chemicals We Eat* (American Heritage Press, 1971). Argues that commercial food additives are as safe as possible; that many "natural" foods naturally contain more dangerous chemicals than manufactured foods do.

F. Bodin and C. F. Cheinisse, *Poisons* (World University Library, 1970). Excellent overview of the many industrial and synthetic chemicals that can poison people today.

Dr. Thomas D. Brock, *The Biology of Microorganisms* (Prentice-Hall, 1974). A very readable textbook on microbes that make toxins and what these toxins do to the human body.

Robin Clarke, *The Silent Weapons* (McKay, 1968). An incisive look at what poisons have been used in warfare up to now.

Hubert Creekmore, *Daffodils Are Dangerous* (Walker and Co., 1966). All about poisonous plants.

John Glaister, *The Power of Poison* (Morrow, 1955). Some fascinating and notorious cases of murder by poison.

Bruce W. Halstead, *Poisonous and Venomous Marine Animals of the World* (U. S. Government Printing Office, 1965). An enormous three-volume work on toxic marine animals throughout the world, but readable and with many colored photos. Updated volumes are expected in the near future.

Beatrice Trum Hunter, *Consumer Beware! Your Food and What's Been Done to It* (Simon & Schuster, 1971). A well researched look at the many poisons and doubtful chemicals added to foods at all stages, and the double-talk that protects these practices.

———, *Food Additives and Federal Policy: The Mirage of Safety* (Scribner's, 1976). A documented description of government laxity in its testing and approval of food additives.

Michael F. Jacobson, *Eater's Digest: The Consumer's Factbook of Food Additives* (Doubleday, 1972). Singles out the most widespread, most useful, most questionable additives.

John M. Kingsbury, *Deadly Harvest* (Holt, Rinehart and Winston, 1965). Historical and modern perspective on poisonous plants and what they do to people.

Ibert and Eleanor Mellan, *Dictionary of Poisons* (Philosophical Library, 1956). A historical look at biological and nonbiological poisons and their effects on people.

Magazine Articles

"Chemical and Biological Weapons," *Scientific American*, May 1970

"Chemical Warfare," *Senior Scholastic*, January 12, 1970

"Chemical Warfare—the Initial Horror," *New Scientist* (London), April 17, 1975

"Chemical Warfare—the Peacetime Legacy," *New Scientist* (London), April 24, 1975

"Combating the Red Tide," *Science News*, August 2, 1975

"How to Deal with Poisonings," *Medical World News*, March 22, 1976

"Phosphorus Poisoning in Children," *Journal of the American Medical Association*, March 29, 1976

"Poisons—Tools of Science," *Science World* (Scholastic Magazines), May 2, 1974

"Snakebite!" *Today's Health*, December 1973

"Some Foods Must Be Cooked," *Prevention*, July 1974

"Watch Out for Food Poisoning," *Changing Times*, August 1975

Index